LEARNING STYLES AND THE NURSING PROFESSION

LEARNING STYLES AND THE NURSING PROFESSION

Rita Dunn

and

Shirley A. Griggs

Editors

St. John's University, New York

NLN Press • New York
Pub. No. 14-7718

The figure used on the chapter openers was designed by
Dr. Rita Dunn & Dr. Kenneth Dunn (1989).

Copyright © 1998
National League for Nursing
350 Hudson Street, New York, NY 10014

The views expressed in this book reflect those of the
authors and do not necessarily reflect the official views
of the National League for Nursing.

Library of Congress Cataloging-in-Publication Data

Learning styles and the nursing profession / Rita Dunn and Shirley A.
Griggs, editors.
     p.   cm.
   Includes bibliographical references and index.
   ISBN 0-88737-771-8
   1. Nursing—Study and teaching.   2. Learning, Psychology of.
3. Cognitive styles.   I. Dunn, Rita Stafford 1930–   .   II. Griggs,
Shirley A.
   [DNLM: 1. Education, Nursing—methods.   2. Learning.   3. Teaching—
methods.   WY 18 L4382 1998]   .
   RT73.L382   1998
   610.73′071—dc21
   DNLM/DLC
   for Library of Congress   97-49117
                                                                    CIP

This book was set in Bembo by Publications Development Company, Crockett, Texas. The
designer was Allan Graubard, and the editor was Maryan Malone. The printer was Clarkwood
Corp. The cover was designed by Lauren Stevens.

Printed in the United States of America.

About the Authors

Rita Dunn, EdD, MA, is Professor, Division of Administrative and Instructional Leadership, and Director of the Center for the Study of Learning and Teaching Styles, St. John's University, New York. She is author/co-author of textbooks and published articles and is the recipient of many professional research awards.

Shirley A. Griggs, EdD, MA, is professor and coordinator of counseling, Division of Human Services and Counseling, St. John's University, New York.

Rose Lefkowitz, MPA, RRA, is Associate Professor, State University of New York's Health Science Center at Brooklyn College of Health-Related Professions. She is a St. John's University Instructional Leadership doctoral candidate and an article and book author.

Dorothy Griggs, MSN, RN, is Assistant Professor, McAuley School of Nursing, University of Detroit-Mercy, Detroit, Michigan.

Joyce Miller, EdD, MM, RDMS, is clinical assistant professor and chairperson of the Diagnostic Imaging Program, College of Health Related Professions, State University of New York Health Science Center in Brooklyn. Dr. Miller is a St. John's University Instructional Leadership graduate and the author of many published articles.

Joyce Morse, MA, RNC, PNP, FAAMR, is Director, Children Services Division, Matheny School and Hospital, Peapack, New Jersey. She is a prolific writer for health professions journals and has had several books published.

Elizabeth A. Van Wynen, MA, RN, CNA, is Instructor of Nursing, Dominican College, Orangeburg, New York. She is a doctoral candidate in St. John's University's Instructional Leadership Program and has had several articles published on applications of learning styles to nursing.

Joan Oberer, MEd, is Principal, Marshall Hill Elementary School, West Milford, New Jersey. She is a doctoral candidate in St. John's University's Instructional Leadership Program.

Joanne Dobbins, MEd, is Director of Remediation Enrichment, St. Stephens–St. Edward Elementary School, Warwick, New York. She is a doctoral candidate in St. John's University's Instructional Leadership Program.

Diane Mitchell, MEd, is Special Education teacher, Clarkstown High School South, West Nyack, New York. She is a doctoral candidate in St. John's University's Instructional Leadership Program.

Lauren E. O'Hare, MSN, RN, is a five-year veteran of full-time nursing instruction at Wagner College, Staten Island, New York. She teaches sophomore, junior, and senior levels of adult health, theory, and clinical supervision.

Contents

Introduction

Learning Styles and the Nursing Profession

Dorothy B. Griggs, MSN, RN

Shirley A. Griggs, EdD, MA

P erusal of the literature in the health professions over the past 20 years indicates a recognition of the importance of the learning-style construct. Using Med Line, Dissertation Abstracts International, Educational Information Resource Center, Compact Disc-Read Only Memory, Cumulative Index to Nursing and Allied Literature, and Psychological Abstracts between 1978 and 1997, a literature search identified 78 studies that were conducted on learning styles in the fields of nursing ($n = 53$), medicine ($n = 15$), dentistry ($n = 4$), medical technology ($n = 1$), and dental hygiene ($n = 1$). The preponderance of these studies were at the undergraduate level in schools of nursing.

In these studies, the learning style instrument most frequently used was Kolb's Learning Style Inventory (1976) ($n = 33$), followed by Dunn, Dunn, and Price's PEPS (1982) ($n = 6$), Gregorc's Style Delineator (1982) ($n = 5$), the Myers-Briggs Type Indicator (1962) ($n = 5$), Schmeck's Inventory of Learning Processes (1977) ($n = 3$), Zenhausern's Hemispheric Preference Test ($n = 3$), Canfield's Learning Style Inventory (1976) ($n = 3$), and other miscellaneous instruments. The vast majority of these studies were correlational in design ($n = 56$), exploring the learning-style differences between traditional versus nontraditional nursing students, freshmen versus seniors, instructors versus students, or correlates of students at risk of terminating their studies. The next most frequently employed design was predictive ($n = 7$), with researchers attempting to identify the learning-style characteristics of high achievers or those in various nursing or medical specialties. Some studies addressed the validity and reliability of different learning-style instruments with nursing or medical students ($n = 2$). Additional studies were literature reviews ($n = 2$) or application studies ($n = 2$) in which learning-style characteristics were related to patient education or career specialty choices. It was disappointing to find few experimental studies ($n = 6$) that addressed the effects of matching various instructional modes to differing learning-style patterns among students (Griggs, Griggs, Dunn, & Ingham, 1994).

Although researchers in the health professions show evidence of an interest in the learning styles of students in the preprofessional level, there seems to be a mind-set that, once the learning style of nursing, medical, or dental students is diagnosed, there is *one best* instructional mode for these students. For example, the finding that the majority of dental students were concrete sequential learners (using Gregorc's *Style Delineator*) led researchers to conclude that order, direct, step-by-step instruction and hands-on experiences are important in the education of this entire population. What seems to be lacking in much of the research, however, is an emphasis on the concept of *individual differences* and that students in the health professions evidence a wide variety of learning-style preferences that need to be accommodated in the instructional process.

This book is designed for health professionals in nursing as well as dentistry, diagnostic medical sonography, medicine, and other related specialties in preprofessional and inservice education. It explains how responding to students' learning styles is beneficial to both the learning and teaching process and provides practical examples of how health professionals implement learning-style strategies.

The following guidelines are presented to assist you in experimenting with learning-style strategies:

1. Identify a learning-style assessment instrument that is appropriate for an adult population and also evidences strong reliability and validity (Curry, 1987; DeCoux, 1990; LaMothe et al., 1991).

2. Administer the instrument that meets the above criteria to the population of health-professionals whose learning styles you want to identify. In many areas, learning-style assessment is mandated by law. The agency that services persons with a disability (Vocational and Educational Services for Individuals with Disabilities [VESID])

requires learning-style identification for all rehabilitation clients. Similarly, the New York State Department of Education specifies that educators must consider students' individual learning styles by accommodating them instructionally.

3. Provide an interpretation of the results of the learning-style assessment to each student and explain his or her individual style strengths. Nelson and others (1993) reported that knowledge of learning-style preferences significantly increased community college students' achievement and reduced the drop-out rate.

4. Provide students with individual "prescriptions" for studying and doing homework through their learning-style strengths (Dunn & Klavas, 1987). Lenehan and others (1994) found that these homework guides based on students' unique learning-style patterns statistically increased undergraduate nurses' science grades and overall grade-point averages and significantly reduced their anxiety and anger scores compared to those of nursing students who had been provided conventional study-skill guidelines.

5. Accommodate students' varied perceptual preferences while teaching. For example, lecture, encourage small-group discussions, and recommend audiotapes, audiodiscs, records, and videocassettes for auditory learners. Recommend charts, graphics, paradigms, videocassettes, and films in addition to books for visual learners. Suggest computer-assisted instruction, note taking, mapping, and illustrating for the retention of tactual learners, and experiential activities, role playing, pantomime, and floor games for kinesthetic learners.

6. Permit accommodations for different acoustical, illumination, and seating preferences in each classroom in which you teach. Individuals vary greatly in their need for quiet versus sound, bright light versus low light, and formal versus informal seating while concentrating. Students' awareness of their strengths and teachers' tolerance go a long way toward facilitating learning.

7. In addition to teacher-directed lessons, occasionally use small-group and individualized instructional approaches to help self-teaching and peer-oriented students enjoy learning.

8. If you find that your class is comprised of many global, rather than analytic processors, try beginning each lesson with an overview of the topic and, if possible, humorous examples of how the content relates to your students' lives. If this aspect of learning style is particularly interesting, see Chapter 3.

The major tenet of learning-style theory is practically oriented and conceptually concise. Accommodating students' learning-style preferences and strengths through compatible instructional interventions results in increased academic achievement. This tenet was supported by a meta-analytic study of 36 quality experimental studies based on the Dunn and Dunn model with a database of 3,181 participants that yielded a weighted effect size value of .353 (Sullivan, 1993). Referring to the standard normal curve, this finding suggests that students whose learning styles are accommodated can be expected to achieve 75 percent of a standard deviation higher than students whose learning styles are not accommodated. This finding indicates that matching students' learning-style preferences with educational interventions compatible with those characteristics is beneficial to their academic achievement. Selected variables were studied in this meta-analysis and revealed the following findings:

1. Accommodating students' physiological preferences has a greater impact than addressing their emotional, environmental, sociological, or combined preferences.

2. Students with strong learning-style preferences showed greater academic gains as a result of congruent instructional interventions than those who had mixed or moderate preferences.

3. College and adult learners showed greater gains than elementary or secondary school learners.

4. Examination of socioeconomic status indicated that middle-class students were more responsive to learning-style accommodations than were students in other socioeconomic categories.

5. Academic-level moderators indicated that average students were more responsive to learning-style accommodations than were high, low, or mixed-achieving groups of students.

6. Instructional interventions that were conducted for more than one year showed stronger results than those conducted for several days, weeks, or months (Dunn, Griggs, Olson, Gorman, & Beasley, 1995).

To summarize, making long-term provisions for the learning-style preferences of students will have the greater impact on college and adult, middle-class, average-achieving persons with strong preferences in the physiological domain. Certainly, many individuals preparing in or working for health profession careers fit this profile.

This book's contributors are healthcare educators who identify and describe instructional interventions that accommodate students' learning-style strengths in their specialty areas. The content of subsequent chapters is summarized as follows:

In Chapter 1, Dunn and Griggs overview the Dunn and Dunn Learning-Style Model and compare it with other models. They synthesize the extensive research base that serves as the cornerstone of the model and elaborate on which learning-style identification instruments provide the type of student information likely to increase achievement.

In Chapter 2, Morse, Oberer, Dobbins, and Mitchell describe a plan for conducting in-service education for nurses based on the participants' learning-style preferences. This chapter is written with different prescriptions for learning the content of the material based on the perceptual strengths of the reader. Visual, auditory, tactual, and kinesthetic learners are directed to learn the material through their personal perceptual preference. The contrasting styles of global versus analytic learners are identified and described through two very different approaches used by nurses when studying for certification in critical care. Instructional techniques that accommodate various nurses' preferences for learning in small groups are described, including circle of knowledge, team learning, and brainstorming. Based on their perceived learning-style profiles, readers are instructed on how to teach themselves with techniques that complement their individual preferences.

In Chapter 3, the learning-style characteristics of global and analytic processors are identified by Van Wynen. She illustrates how the Dunn and Dunn Learning-Style Model has been applied successfully in a senior-level baccalaureate nursing course, "Leadership and Management of Patient Care."

In Chapter 4, Lefkowitz explains how Edna Huffman's widely used textbook in the field of health information has been translated into programmed learning sequences (PLS) designed to accommodate varied perceptual strengths and both global and analytic processing styles.

In Chapter 5, Miller addresses the processes of applying learning-style instructional techniques to the preparation of diagnostic medical sonography baccalaureate students by beginning with individual counseling sessions to interpret their assessment results. Several programmed learning sequences were developed for units on the anatomy of the brain, normal renal ultrasound, and pathology in various body systems using both a booktype format and interactive CD ROM multimedia. The results of an experimental study contrasting how medical students with different learning styles performed in traditional lectures versus the book PLS versus the computer PLS format may be surprising.

These healthcare educators developed Chapters 2 through 5 based on their classroom experiences with the Dunn and Dunn Learning-Style Model. We believe that their descriptions will entice you into identifying the learning styles of your students and experimenting with some of the suggested approaches that worked so well for them.

Chapter 1

Learning Styles: Link Between Teaching and Learning

Rita Dunn, EdD, MA

Shirley A. Griggs, EdD, MA

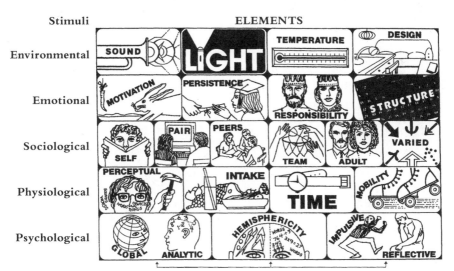

Stimuli	ELEMENTS			
Environmental	SOUND	LiGHT	TEMPERATURE	DESIGN
Emotional	MOTIVATION	PERSISTENCE	RESPONSIBILITY	STRUCTURE
Sociological	SELF	PAIR	PEERS / TEAM / ADULT	VARIED
Physiological	PERCEPTUAL	INTAKE	TIME	MOBILITY
Psychological	GLOBAL / ANALYTIC	HEMISPHERICITY	IMPULSIVE	REFLECTIVE

Simultaneous or Successive Processing

Knowledge about learning styles and brain behavior is a fundamental new tool. . . . It provides a deeper and more profound view of the learner than previously perceived, and is part of a basic framework upon which a sounder theory and practice of learning and instruction may be built.

Keefe, 1982, Foreword

THE DUNN AND DUNN LEARNING-STYLE MODEL

The widely used Dunn and Dunn (1972, 1975, 1978, 1992, 1993) Learning-Style Model is based on the theory that each person has biologically and developmentally imposed characteristics that respond either positively or negatively to a variety of environmental, emotional, sociological, physiological, cognitive, and instructional variables. Recognition and response to such variables is a means to enhance student learning.

Learning style, as the Dunns describe it, is the way individuals begin to concentrate on, process, internalize, and remember *new and difficult academic information or skills.* They identify style by individuals' reactions to learning: (a) in their immediate instructional environment (sound, light, temperature, design); (b) emotionally (motivation, persistence, responsibility, structure); (c) sociologically (learning alone, with peers, with either a collegial or authoritative adult, and/or with a variety of approaches as opposed to patterns or routines); (d) physiologically (auditory, visual, tactual, and/or kinesthetic perceptual preferences, time-of-day energy levels,

11

food intake, and mobility needs); and (e) global versus analytic processing (see Figure on page 9).

Higher Education Research with the Dunn and Dunn Model

Many researchers have identified college students' learning styles with instruments, and especially those related to the Dunn and Dunn Model.
They have experimented with instructional treatments for studying course
assignments based on individuals' preferences. Generally, significantly
higher achievement was reported when the studying strategies were congruent, rather than incongruent, with each student's identified learning
style in courses in anatomy (Cook, 1989; Lenehan, Dunn, Ingham, Murray, & Signer, 1994; Miller, 1997), bacteriology (Lenehan et al., 1994),
marketing (Dunn, Deckinger, Withers, & Katzenstein, 1990), mathematics (Dunn, Bruno, Sklar, Zenhausern, & Beaudry, 1990), physiology
(Lenehan et al., 1994), sonography (Miller, 1997), across subjects (Clark-
Thayer, 1987, 1988; Mickler & Zippert, 1987), and in grade-point averages (Lenehan et al., 1994; Nelson et al., 1993).

For example, Clark-Thayer (1987) identified underachieving, college
freshmen's learning styles with the Productivity Environmental Preference Survey (PEPS) (Dunn, Dunn, & Price, 1982, 1989). She assigned
trained tutors to teach freshmen to study with strategies that responded to
their learning-style preferences. Students' achievement increased significantly ($p > .01$) when they studied with strategies congruent, rather than
incongruent, with their learning-style preferences. In a subsequent study,
Clark-Thayer (1988) described students' improved attitudes toward course
content after they learned to study with congruent strategies.

Dunn, Bruno, et al. (1990) identified the processing styles of 1,000
minority college students in remedial mathematics classes with the
PEPS. The majority of these students were global processors; the textbook assigned to that class was written in a step-by-step analytic style in

which procedures were itemized but no direct application was provided. The researchers revised every other chapter in the textbook to reflect global processing but kept intact the alternate analytic chapters. Students were required to study all the chapters independently. Requiring students to learn from alternative global and analytic math chapters without direct teacher instruction (a) eliminated what could have become an intervening variable of teaching style and (b) resulted in significantly higher test scores ($p < .001$) on the chapters that matched, rather than mismatched, individuals' global versus analytic preferences.

Instead of focusing on a single element of learning style, such as global versus analytic preferences, Nelson et al. (1993) identified individual freshmen's learning styles with the PEPS and provided directions for studying with complementary strategies. The matched prescriptions significantly impacted student achievement ($p > .01$) and retention ($p > .01$), and the drop-out rate was reduced to 20 percent in contrast to the usual rate of 39 percent.

Cook (1989), Dunn, Deckinger, et al. (1990) and Mickler and Zippert (1987) also identified students' learning styles with the PEPS and revealed significant improvement ($p > .01$) when learners were made aware of their learning styles and studied accordingly. These researchers showed college students how to capitalize on their learning-style preferences to study for specific college courses, whereas Nelson et al. (1993) evaluated the effectiveness of learning-style applications in a formal academic advisement program, and Clark-Thayer (1987) provided trained tutors in a campus learning center.

The efficacy of responding to individuals' learning styles was also examined by Miller (1997) in an urban college of allied health professions in a large state university. The experimental sample consisted of junior and senior college students enrolled in Sonography 1 ($n = 23$) and Cross-Sectional Anatomy ($n = 17$). The experiment consisted of alternating traditional professorial lectures reinforced with visuals and readings and counterbalanced by a booktype programmed learning sequence (PLS) as designed by Dunn and Dunn (1993), counterbalanced by a computer version of the same kind of PLS. Individual learning-style assessments were generated with the PEPS (Dunn, Dunn, & Price, 1982, 1989).

Most students' achievement test scores were statistically higher (p < .001) with the book and computer forms of the PLS than with traditional teaching in both anatomy and sonography. The effect size in the former was .63, indicating only a moderate effect, but the effect size in sonography was 1.42, indicating a very strong difference between the two methodologies. However, clear relationships were evidenced between the results and the students' learning-style preferences. For example, students who preferred learning:

1. With the book PLS, preferred quiet while concentrating and did not perform as well in the traditional lessons or with the computer-generated PLS, which generated noise;

2. Alone, performed best with the book PLS and significantly less well when required to concentrate with others nearby—as occurs in a classroom or in a computer lab;

3. With an authoritative figure present, performed best in the traditional lessons; and

4. In learning-style responsive treatments, attained statistically higher attitude scores.

In a study directly related to nursing, Lenehan et al., (1994) used the Learning Style Inventory (Dunn, Dunn, & Price, 1989) to identify the learning styles of 203 undergraduate nursing majors. Students in two required science courses—Anatomy and Physiology ($n = 134$) and Bacteriology ($n = 69$)—were randomly selected from a population of 296 first-time, full-time, predominantly female, freshmen nursing and transfer students. They then were randomly assigned to either an experimental or a control group.

Students in the experimental group were shown how to study by capitalizing on their identified learning-style preferences. All students were shown how to study with conventional study-skill guidelines, tutoring, and advisement assistance. These students achieved statistically higher science grades *and* grade-point averages than students in the control group, suggesting that homework prescriptions for use in one subject may positively affect grades in other subjects.

In addition, the experimental group evidenced significantly lower anxiety and anger scores on the State-Trait Personality Inventory (Spielberger et al., 1979) and higher curiosity about science as the term progressed. At the semester's end, students in the control group were significantly more anxious about and angry with their science course(s) than those in the experimental group, and their curiosity about science had declined. Thus, using learning-style responsive strategies to prepare baccalaureate nursing students, either for their course work or to take the National Licensing Examination, may be the missing link between faculty teaching and student academic success.

HOW DO PEOPLE'S LEARNING STYLES DIFFER?

Learning styles vary with (a) age (Dunn & Griggs, 1995; Price, 1980), (b) achievement level (Milgram, Dunn, & Price, 1993), (c) gender, (d) culture (Dunn & Griggs, 1995; Milgram, Dunn, & Price, 1993), and (e) global versus analytic brain processing (Dunn, Bruno, et al., 1990; Dunn, Cavanaugh, Eberle, & Zenhausern, 1982). In a review of multiculturally diverse students in many nations, Dunn and Griggs (1995) reported different styles within each group and that there seemed to be more within- than between-group distinctions. For example, in each family, the mother and father tend to have diametrically opposite learning styles, their first two offspring rarely learned similarly.

Four variables significantly differ between groups and among individuals within the same group:

1. *High versus low academic achievement:* Although many gifted students learn differently from each other and underachievers have many different learning styles, gifted and underachieving students have statistically different learning styles and do not learn well with the same methods. Conversely, gifted students in nine diverse cultures—with talent in either athletics, art, dance, leadership, literature, mathematics, or music—evidenced learning-style characteristics similar to other students with the same talent (Milgram et al., 1993).

2. *Gender:* Males and females often learn differently. Males tend to be more visual, tactual, and kinesthetic, and need mobility in an informal environment. Males also are more nonconforming and peer-motivated than their female counterparts (Dunn & Dunn, 1992, 1993; Dunn & Griggs, 1995).

    Females, more so than males, tend to be auditory, conforming, authority-oriented, and better able to sit passively in conventional classroom desks and chairs. Females also tend to need significantly more quiet while learning (Pizzo, Dunn, & Dunn, 1990), and they are more parent- and self-motivated than males (Marcus, 1977).

3. *Age:* Learning styles change the longer students remain in school and continue to change as they grow older (Dunn & Griggs, 1995; Price, 1980). Sociological preferences for learning alone, with an authoritative versus a collegial teacher and with routines as opposed to preferring a variety of social approaches, develop over time, change with age and maturity, and are developmental. Motivation, responsibility (conformity versus nonconformity), and internal versus external structure also are developmental (Thies, 1979).

    Less than 25 percent of college students are auditory learners—able to remember approximately 75 percent of the new and difficult information they listen to during a 40- to 50-minute period. Less than 40 percent are visual learners—able to remember approximately 75 percent of what they read during a 40- to 50-minute period. Although auditory and visual modalities develop with age, many adult males are neither auditory nor visual learners, remaining only tactual or kinesthetic learners throughout their lives (Ingham, 1991).

4. *How individuals process new and difficult information:* Studies of global and analytic processors revealed that relationships exist among processing styles and environmental, emotional, sociological, and/or physiological learning-style preferences, which often were clustered. For example, learning persistently (with few or no intermissions), in a quiet, well-lit, formal setting with little or no intake often correlated with being an analytic processor. Learning with intermittent periods of concentration and relaxation, in soft lighting and with music or other sounds while seated informally and snacking, correlated with a highly global processing style (Cody 1983; Dunn, Bruno, et al., 1990; Dunn et al., 1982). Although global students often preferred learning tactually and with peers (Jarsonbeck, 1984), no clear perceptual or social pattern was revealed among analytics.

Other Learning-Style Models

Examination of various learning-style definitions revealed that despite differences in terminology, the models themselves overlapped (Dunn, DeBello, Brennan, Krimsky, & Murrain, 1981). For example, motivation and sociological traits were addressed by Canfield and Lafferty (1976), Dunn and Dunn (1978), Gregorc (1982), Hill (1971), and Ramirez and Castenada (1974). Structure was included in the models of Canfield and Lafferty, Dunn and Dunn, Gregorc, Hill, Hunt, and Ramirez and Castenada and, with the exception of Ramirez and Castenada, these researchers and Kolb (1976) acknowledged perception as a learning-style variable. Brain processing was addressed by Canfield and Lafferty, Dunn and Dunn, Gregorc, Hill, Kolb, Ramirez and Castenada, and Schmeck (1977).

Differences also exist among these models. Canfield and Lafferty addressed goal setting; whereas, two decades ago, the Dunns described intake, sound, light, temperature, seating, mobility, variety versus routine preferences, and time-of-day energy levels. The Dunns also differentiated among learning alone, in pairs, as part of a team, with peers, with collegial versus authoritative adults, and with variety versus routines and patterns. And, well in advance of current interest in multiculturalism, both the Hill and Ramirez and Castenada models included culture in their respective frameworks. During the mid-1980s when the National Association of Secondary School Principals' model (NASSP) (Keefe, Languis, Letteri, & Dunn, 1986) was released, its variables essentially paralleled those in the Dunns' model and McCarthy's 4 MAT system essentially parallels Gregorc's and Kolb's categories (DeBello, 1990).

LEARNING-STYLE RESEARCH

The research on learning styles is uneven across models. The NASSP model is comparatively young (1986); in contrast, the Dunn and Dunn model has been developing since the late 1960s. DeBello (1990) noted that the Dunn and Dunn and Hunt, Kolb, and Schmeck models were developed at universities by graduate faculty and doctoral students; the NASSP model was designed under the auspices of the nation's largest secondary school association; some models are promulgated by commercial firms with only minimal research documentation.

DeBello described some models as narrow in focus with only one or two variables on a bipolar continuum, whereas the Dunn and Dunn, Hill, and NASSP models are comprehensive, each requiring analysis of 20 or more variables. DeBello also challenged the learning-style nomenclature of certain models. Myers-Briggs (1962) is essentially a personality index and 4 MAT is a lesson-plan design that prescribes teaching all students in the same class with the same resources, in the same sequence, in the same way, at the same time, and for the same amount of time. Finally, the quality of learning-styles research varies from model to model and from study to study. In comparison, the literature reports more than 500 studies with the Dunn and Dunn Learning-Style Model by researchers at more than 100 different colleges and universities (*Research on the Dunn and Dunn Model,* 1997).

INSTRUMENTS FOR IDENTIFYING
LEARNING STYLE

Although the concept of individual differences appears to have the nursing profession's fundamental support, much of the research concerning matching instructional methods to nurses' styles has not revealed significant findings (DeCoux, 1990; Laschinger & Bass, 1984). In contrast, similar studies in elementary, secondary, and college classes have yielded significantly increased achievement, improved attitudes toward instruction, and better discipline (St. John's University, Center for the Study of Learning and Teaching Styles, 1997). Comparisons of the latter studies with those conducted with nurses revealed the use of very different instruments to identify individuals' learning styles.

Many learning-style instruments purport to measure individual learning styles (DeBello, 1990). Examination of those considered reliable and valid by Curry (1987) revealed that the instruments used in the nursing studies—that repeatedly failed to impact instructional improvement when apparently complementing nurses' styles—were different from the instruments used in studies in which significant gains were consistently reported. Apparently different instruments yielded different results. Thus, it is important to consider how these instruments differ and whether their differences might account for the disparate results.

Curry's Onion Model of Learning and Cognitive Style

Curry (1987) conceived a theoretical framework in which learning-style models and their related instruments could be examined. Her "onion model" encompassed approximately 25 learning-style instruments and identified four layers:

1. *Personality dimensions*—the core of the onion—were relatively stable traits of basic personality, such as those measured by the Myers-Briggs Type Indicator (1962);

2. *Information-processing models*—the next layer—addressed the individual's preferred intellectual approach to assimilating information, as operationalized in Kolb's (1976) Learning Style Inventory and Schmeck's (1977) Inventory of Learning Processes;

3. *Social interaction models* addressed *how* students functioned in the classroom, as measured by Witkin's (1971) Embedded Figures Test that identified field-dependent versus field-independent learners; and

4. *Multidimensional* and *instructional preferences models* as assessed by Dunn, Dunn, and Price's Productivity Environmental Preference Survey (PEPS) (1982, 1989) for mature adults and versions of their Learning Style Inventory for grades 3 through 12 encompass all of

the constructs of the three previous layers to comprehensively assess between 21 and 23 elements of learning style. The number of elements assessed vary with the form of the instrument and is based on the age of the students for which it is deemed appropriate.

Curry proposed that (a) each of the layers represented separate and discrete constructs, (b) very few instruments assessed more than one level, and (c) the PEPS was one of the few instruments with good reliability and validity. Curry's position was endorsed by DeCoux, (1990) who observed that the innumerable learning-style instruments were strikingly dissimilar and that the theoretical constructs on which they were based contained only tenuous connections.

In contrast, Griggs (1993) reported that the Dunn and Dunn model was multidimensional and thus held promise for the application of learning styles to the education of health professionals. Apropos of nursing, Griggs' position had been supported by LaMothe et al.'s (1991) establishment of reliability of the PEPS based on a sample of 443 baccalaureate nursing students.

Experimental Studies in the Health Professions

Three experimental studies examined the impact of accommodating nursing students' *individual* leaning styles. Billings and Cobb (1992) studied the major effects of learning-style preferences, attitudes, and grade-point averages on the learning achievement of student nurses when using computer-assisted, interactive videodisc instruction. Results indicated that student GPA was positively correlated with individual motivation and responsibility scores; that is, students with higher grade-point averages were significantly more motivated and responsible than students with lower grade-point averages.

Buell and Buell (1987) explored the relationship of the perceptual preferences of 61 teachers, 31 nurses, and their 8 instructors' perceptual preferences to the participants' assessed satisfaction and knowledge following in-service training sessions. Findings revealed that (a) a majority of participants had various perceptual preferences that influenced their learning; (b) preferences were significantly related to the satisfaction participants reported with the format, content, and presenter of the sessions; and (c) presenters' sessions reflected their own perceptual preferences.

Finally, Lenehan and others (1994) found that science achievement scores, overall grade-point average, and curiosity about learning required science were significantly higher, and anxiety and anger were significantly lower, among baccalaureate nursing students who were taught how to study by capitalizing on their individual learning-style preferences, as compared with students who were taught how to study with conventional study-skills applications.

LEARNING STYLE AND INSTRUCTIONAL PREFERENCE

Instructional preference describes the ways in which individuals concentrate on and remember new and difficult material. Instructional preference is directly related to the methods, resources, or approaches students favor. The Myers-Briggs Type Indicator (1962) focuses on personality dimensions, Kolb's Learning Style Inventory (1976) and Schmeck's Inventory of Learning Processes (1977) focus on information processing, and Witkin's Embedded Figures Test (1977) focuses on social interaction dimensions. Each of these test a separate variable related to how individuals learn. In contrast, Dunn, Dunn, and Price's Productivity Environmental Preference Survey (PEPS) (1982) focuses on multiple learning-style variables and yields information concerning 23 environmental, personality, social interaction, physiological, and global versus analytic processing preferences obtained from correlations in individual PEPS printouts.

As previously reported, experimental research conducted with the PEPS revealed significantly increased undergraduate college student achievement in matched versus mismatched treatments (Cook, 1989; Dunn, Bruno, et al., 1990; Ingham, 1990; Mickler & Zippert, 1987; Nelson, Dunn, et al., 1993; Lenehan et al., 1994). Finally, a metaanalysis of 36 quality experimental studies conducted with the Dunn and Dunn model at 13 universities during 1980–1990 revealed that students whose learning styles are accommodated can be expected to achieve 75 percent of a standard deviation higher than students whose learning styles are not accommodated (Dunn et al., 1995). Thus, matching students' learning styles with educational interventions compatible with those characteristics is beneficial to their academic achievement.

SUMMARY

Chapter 1 provided an introduction to learning styles and reviewed selected research with the Dunn and Dunn model. Succeeding chapters describe applications of that model as experienced by successful health profession practitioners.

CHAPTER 2

Understanding Learning Styles: Implications for In-Service Educators

Joyce S. Morse, MA, RNC, PNP, FAAMR

Joan Oberer, M Ed

Jo-Anne Dobbins, M Ed

Diane Mitchell, M Ed

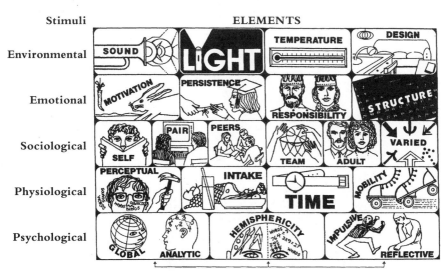

It is 5:00 P.M. on a Thursday evening. As I look around the classroom, I notice that most of the 15 registered nurses in the IV certification course appear weary. Despite the fact that most of them worked the 7 A.M. to 3 P.M. shift and have families waiting for them at home, they are making a valiant effort to remain alert. After we take a break for a snack, the class reconvenes and we divide into two groups. We then use a small-group technique called *circle of knowledge* to identify types and characteristics of IV solutions. The group is almost magically revitalized. The students leave, albeit reluctantly, almost 20 minutes past the scheduled end of class time!

What occurred after the break was not a miracle. It demonstrated a teaching approach that appealed to the majority of the students in the class. Understanding the concept of learning styles assists in-service educators to optimize the learning experience for each participant. This chapter discusses learning styles, how to assess the learning styles of registered nurse participants in in-service education programs, and the implications of using a learning-styles approach.

DEFINITION

Dunn and Dunn define *learning style* as a "biological and developmental set of personal characteristics that makes the identical instruction effective for some students and ineffective for others" (Dunn & Dunn, 1993, p. 5). Their Learning-Style Model is based on two theories of learning: cognitive style theory and brain lateralization. Many variables impact on the learning style of each person. The learning style of the individual

27

explains how that person is able to learn new and difficult information, concentrate, understand, and retain it. Learning styles involve four perceptual strengths, according to Dunn and Dunn (1993), they are:

1. Visual (30–40% of learners)

2. Auditory (20–30% of learners)

3. Tactual (20–25% of learners)

4. Kinesthetic (20–25% of learners)

Most students learn through one of two processing styles. They are either *global* or *analytic* learners. In-service educators are faced with the challenge of providing both mandatory and optional class materials to a very diverse population. Some learners are novices in the field of nursing while others may have had many years of experience. Using a learning-style model facilitates success for each learner.

HOW TO READ THIS CHAPTER

As you read this chapter, you will learn more about the perceptual and processing preferences involved in learning styles. Most teaching strategies engage only *one* perceptual strength.

- If you are a *visual learner,* you will respond well to this chapter because it contains text and graphics.

- *Auditory learners:* Try reading this chapter aloud or have someone read it to you.

- *Tactual learners:* Use a highlighter, write notes all over this chapter, or even cut the relevant information out and paste it on index cards.

- *Kinesthetic learners:* Walk around while reading, but watch out for obstacles!

Understanding Instructional Preferences

During the 1960s and 1970s, Letteri (1985) labeled learners as field dependent and field independent. An example of a field-dependent learner
is a global-type person. The RN who enjoys working from case studies
is usually a field-dependent learner. This is the person who likes to peruse
a subject, overlooking the details to get the big picture. Field-independent
learners are more analytical. They *must* know the details before they can
do anything with information (Letteri, 1985). As research about learning
styles evolved, Dunn, Cavanaugh, Eberle, and Zenhausern (1982) found
a correlation between learning-style elements and right/left brain dominance. "Left-oriented activators usually are logical, analytical, and sequential—they are successive processors. Right-oriented activators usually
are global, holistic, and intuitive—they are simultaneous processors"
(Freeley & Perrin, 1987, p. 68).

As recently as 1990, Dunn et al. found that when global college students were matched with instructional strategies congruent with their
hemisphericity, they achieved statistically higher performance results.
The research also indicated the existence of a significant relationship
between the students' diagnosed hemisphericity and their learning-style
preference. Research has demonstrated that teachers are able to identify only a few elements of their students' learning styles through ob-
servation; other elements appear to be identifiable through personal
interviewing or the administration of learning-style assessment (Beaty,
1986; Dunn, 1987).

CHARACTERISTICS OF GLOBAL VERSUS ANALYTIC LEARNERS

The global learner is the one whose attention needs to be captured
through the use of short stories, anecdotes, humor, and illustrations.
Global learners need to know what they need to learn and why they

need to learn it. Once they have an understanding of that, they can then concentrate on the details. The other type of learner is the analytic learner. Analytic learners learn best when information is introduced to them step-by-step, fact-by-fact. Analytic learners will listen to all the facts as long as they feel they are heading toward a goal. According to Dunn (1987), approximately 55 percent of adults are global learners, while 28 percent are analytic. The rest can process information comfortably either way, adjusting to circumstances. Most training is designed to teach analytic learners, while the global learners' needs are not addressed (Dunn, 1996). Table 2.1 identifies the preferences of strongly analytic and strongly global students.

Table 2.1   Preferences of Global and Analytic Learners

Strongly Analytic Learners Prefer	Strongly Global Learners Prefer
Quiet while learning	Sound while working
Bright lights	Soft lights
Formal seating (hard chair, desk)	Informal seating (easy chair, bed, carpeting)
Working on a single task until completion, then beginning a new task	Working on several tasks simultaneously with breaks in between
Snacking after completion of a task	Snacking while doing their tasks
Working alone or with an authority figure	Working with peers
Doing things their own way	Following standard directions

Adapted from Dunn & Dunn (1993) *Teaching secondary students through their individual learning style.* Needham Heights, MA: Allyn and Bacon.

UNDERSTANDING LEARNING-STYLE ASSESSMENT TOOLS

In 1994, Griggs, Griggs, Dunn, and Ingham presented a framework for understanding the learning-style needs of nurses as individuals rather than as a group. They used Curry's (1987) review of approximately 25 learning-style assessment tools. Curry had conceived an "onion model" to describe a theoretical framework with four distinct layers. Each layer of the onion was described as a discrete entity because very few of the instruments reviewed assessed more than one level of learning style. The first layer consisted of tools such as the Myers-Briggs Indicator (1962) that assessed stable traits (e.g., personality). The second layer of Curry's model looked at information-processing models like Kolb's Learning Style Inventory (1976). The third layer looked at social interaction models. An example of this type of model would be Witkin's Embedded Figures Test (1971). Curry's fourth layer looked at multidimensional and instructional preference models. The Productivity Environmental Preference Survey (PEPS) of Dunn, Dunn, and Price (1982) fits into this last category.

The PEPS is a measurement of the learning-style preferences of adults, which consists of 100 dichotomous questions that elicit self-diagnostic responses relating to 21 distinct learning-style elements on a 5-point Likert scale (Nelson et al., 1993). The PEPS is one of the few instruments with good reliability and validity (Griggs, Griggs, Dunn, & Ingham, 1994). It focuses on learning-style variables that provide the student and teacher with information about *environmental concerns* (sound, light, temperature, seating design); *emotional dimensions* (motivation, persistence, responsibility [conformity versus nonconformity], and the need for externally imposed structure or the opportunity to do things independently); *social interaction preferences* (learning alone or in a pair, in a small group, as part of a team, or with either collegial or authoritative adults); *physiological preferences* (perceptual strengths, time-of-day energy levels, the need for intake and/or mobility while learning); and *psychological preferences* (global/analytic, right/left, and impulsive/reflective). The figure on page 25 illustrates the variables assessed by the PEPS.

The PEPS was normed using 975 females and 419 males ranging in age from 18 to 65 years. Test, retest reliability for the 20 subscales range from .39 to .87 with 40 percent over .8 correlations (Nelson et al., 1993). Over the past 6 years, the PEPS has demonstrated predictive validity (Buell & Buell, 1987; Dunn et al., 1990; Ingham, 1991; LaMothe et al., 1991).

UNDERSTANDING THE DUNN AND DUNN MODEL

The Dunn and Dunn model is based on the following theoretical assumptions:

1. Most individuals can learn.

2. Instructional environments, resources, and approaches respond to diversified learning-style strengths.

3. Everyone has strengths, but different people have different strengths.

4. Individual instructional preferences exist and can be measured reliably.

5. Given responsive environments, resources, and approaches, students attain statistically higher achievement and attitude test scores in matched, rather than mismatched, treatments.

6. Most teachers can learn to use learning styles as a cornerstone of their instruction.

7. Many students can learn to capitalize on their learning-style strengths when concentrating on new or difficult academic material.

8. The less academically successful the individual, the more important it is to accommodate learning-style preference (Dunn & Dunn, 1993).

USING A LEARNING-STYLE MODEL IN DEVELOPING IN-SERVICE PROGRAMS

To be effective, in-service educators must accommodate students with diverse learning styles in each class. The development of effective learning programs has to take into account variables such as gender and age. Women, in general, tend to be more auditory, self-motivated, conforming, and authority-oriented than their male peers. They are able to sit still in conventional classroom desks and chairs. Women also tend to need significantly more quiet during learning. On the other hand, men tend to be more visual, tactual, and kinesthetic. They need more mobility and an informal environmental design. They tend to be more nonconforming and peer-motivated than their female contemporaries (Marcus, 1977). For both genders, some aspects of learning styles change with age. Older students may require brighter lighting than they did when they were younger. Time-of-day preference is also affected by aging. In-service educators should be aware that approximately 55 percent of adults learn better in the morning (Price, 1980).

Perceptual modalities need to be taken into account by in-service educators as well. Ideally, educators will give learners information in their primary perceptual modality, whether it be visual, auditory, kinesthetic, or tactual. Then the information should be reinforced through their secondary preference. For example, a learner whose primary perceptual modality is visual and whose secondary perceptual strength is kinesthetic could be introduced to information on a chart. Reinforcement could then take place through a kinesthetic activity such as role playing.

Assessment for learning styles as part of an orientation session using the PEPS takes about 20 minutes and does the following:

- Permits students to identify how they prefer to learn and also indicates the degree to which their responses are consistent.

- Provides a computerized summary of each student's preferred learning style.

- Suggests a basis for redesigning the classroom environment to complement many students' needs for sound, quiet, bright or soft light, warmth or coolness, formal or informal seating.

- Describes with whom each student is likely to achieve efficiently. For example, alone, in a pair, with two or more classmates, with others with similar interests, with either a collegial or authoritative teacher and/or with all, none, or any of these possibilities.

- Explains to whom options should be provided and for whom direction and/or structure is appropriate.

- Sequences the perceptual strengths through which individuals should *begin* studying and then *reinforce* new and difficult information.

- Indicates the methods through which students are likely to achieve well.

- Extrapolates information about which students are nonconforming and how to work with them.

- Pinpoints the optimal time of day for learning for each student.

- Identifies the students for whom snacking while learning is an integral part of the process.

- Notes the students who require movement during learning as an integral part of the process.

- Suggests for which students using analytic or global approaches to learning new and difficult material may be important (Dunn & Dunn, 1993).

TEACHING NURSES TO TEACH THEMSELVES

By assisting each learner to understand his or her learning style, the in-service educator can assist each nurse to achieve success in learning activities. To enhance effectiveness as an instructor, introduce the participants in the in-service programs to the concept of learning styles. It is important to stress that everyone has a learning style and strength. These will be as individual and varied as the program participants. When a person knows *how* he or she learns, then that person will be able to learn whatever he or she really wants by creating and using learning materials that teach through their primary strength and reinforce through their secondary strength.

Once individual learning styles have been identified, it is time to teach participants how to create some of the tactual materials that they will use to teach themselves. Students who have an auditory strength learn best when listening to lectures or audiotapes. They can recall 75 percent or more of the material covered in a one-hour lecture. Encourage these students to make audiotapes for future reference.

Visual learners learn best by studying written materials, charts, and diagrams. Many in-service educators already use these materials regularly; but how many actually introduce new and difficult information tactually or kinesthetically for persons with those perceptual strengths? Probably not many, simply because we have not learned how to teach adults using these modalities. The following techniques are designed to allow tactual and kinesthetic learners to use them to teach themselves.

Technique 1: A Flip Chute

How do you introduce lessons tactually? The first suggestion is a *flip chute*. This unique, easily-constructed device can be made in class or at home. Flip chutes are made from half-gallon milk or juice containers. Small question-and-answer cards are designed to be inserted into the upper face of the container. As each card descends on an inner slide, it flips over and emerges through the lower opening with the correct answer on it.

Directions

1. Pull open the top of a half-gallon milk or juice container.

2. Cut the side folds of the top portion down to the top of the container.

3. On the front edge, measure down both (a) 1.5 in. and (b) 2.5 in. Draw lines across the container. Remove that space.

4. Mark up from the bottom (1.5 in. and 2.5 in.). Draw lines across the container. Remove that space.

5. Cut one 5 × 8 index card to measure 6.5 by 3.5 in.

6. Cut a second index card to measure 7.5 by 3.5 in.

7. Fold down .5 in. at both ends of the smaller strip. Fold down at the end of the longer strip.

8. Insert the smaller strip into the bottom opening with the folded edge resting on the upper portion of the bottom opening. Attach it with masking tape.

9. Bring the upper part of the smaller strip over the center section of the carton. Attach it with masking tape.

10. Work the longer strip, one end is folded down and the other end is unfolded. Insert the unfolded end of the longer strip into the bottom opening of the container. Push it into the container until the folded part rests on the bottom part of the container. Attach it with masking tape.

11. Attach the upper edge of the longer strip to the back of the container creating a slide. Secure it with masking tape about .625 in. from the top of the carton.

12. Fold down the top flaps of the container and tape them in place forming a rectangular box.

13. Use small, 2 × 2.5 in. index cards to write the question on one side and the answer upside down on the flip side. Notch each question side at the top right to insure appropriate positioning when the student uses the cards. The flip chutes can be decorated and turned into thematic items or left plain and used with all lessons.

Any information can be put on the cards that are flipped through the chute. Why does this work? Because some students learn best when they physically maneuver or manipulate materials with their hands.

Technique 2: Task Cards

A second strategy for tactual and kinesthetic learners is the use of *task cards*. Put the basic information you want into a question-answer, true-or-false, or matching format. Have the students use two-part cards. Put the question on one part and the corresponding answer on the other. Cut the question apart from the answer and allow the students to put them together like puzzle pieces.

SMALL-GROUP TECHNIQUES

Many participants in in-service activities are stimulated to learn by working within a group. Some participants are able to relax when a group, rather than each of them individually, is responsible for completion of a task. Many small-group techniques can be designed to accommodate varieties in sociological preferences of students. Small-group techniques can be adjusted within the environment to accommodate the elements of light, temperature, design, time intake, and mobility as well. Adults who are peer-oriented, motivated, persistent, and responsible will be able to learn well using these techniques.

Technique 1: Circle of Knowledge

This is a highly motivating technique and provides an ideal opportunity for reinforcing skills. It also can provide a framework for review, allowing the group to focus thinking on one major concept at a time. Procedure: Identify a group of approximately five members. One person is designated as a recorder. The in-service educator identifies the question to be answered by the group and sets a time frame for the response. Usually a 2- to 4-minute time frame is adequate. An example of *circle of knowledge* might be: List as many types of IV solutions that are used in our hospital as you can. If you want to make this a competitive situation, you could have one team play against another team and then score accordingly.

Technique 2: Team Learning

Team learning is an excellent strategy for introducing new or difficult materials. The procedure is to introduce an article or written material containing new information to be learned. A group of four or five participants is assigned to work together. One acts as a recorder. The inservice educator identifies four or five questions that the group has to answer collectively. If there is more than one group working at a time, then each group can contribute one answer to the final session. This technique encourages a lot of interaction among participants.

Technique 3: Brain Storming

Brain storming is a strategy designed to develop multiple answers to a single question through group participation and presentation of alternative and creative solutions to an identified problem. Brain storming not only can be exciting, but also can be stimulating, positive, focused, spontaneous, and creative. It encourages the group to create strategies for ongoing problem solving (Dunn, 1996). A brain-storming group can involve from 5 to 10 participants, with the leader also acting as the recorder.

Technique 4: Case Studies

This commonly-used technique in nursing education is a strategy to stimulate and help develop analytical skills. Usually 4 or 5 participants can spend a considerable amount of time discussing and interpreting short, relevant case study material that teaches something specific. Case studies provide an effective strategy for encouraging critical thinking within the participant's frame of reference. It is an approach that can be stimulating and meaningful if the participants identify with a member of the case study situation. It is a safe, nonthreatening method for participants to enter into the analysis of problem resolution without direct personal consequences.

Additional small-group techniques that nurse in-service educators can use effectively are patient simulation settings, role playing, group analysis, task forces, and study groups or research committees.

CONCLUSION

In-service educators play an important role in assuring the delivery of quality care to consumers. An effective way to engage staff in actively learning the skills necessary to deliver the best possible care in a rapidly changing environment is to optimize each staff member's ability to learn the skills he or she needs.

CHAPTER 3

How Do You Think?:
Two Sides to Every Story

Elizabeth A. Van Wynen, MA, RN, CNA

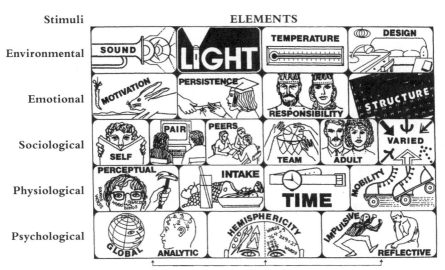

Stimuli   ELEMENTS

Environmental

Emotional

Sociological

Physiological

Psychological

Simultaneous or Successive Processing

The way you think is based on how your brain processes—globally or analytically. Nurse educators must understand the differences involved here to enhance and empower their students' learning abilities. Changing lessons from traditional lecture and note taking to active student involvement, so that students comprehend better than ever before, is an excellent place to start. The purpose of this chapter, then, is to examine two major styles of information processing, identify global and analytic preferences and responsive teaching strategies, and illustrate how these strategies were applied, both to the educator's and the students' advantage, in a baccalaureate nursing course.

GLOBAL AND ANALYTIC PROCESSING

Brains process information differently; individuals perceive, experience, and learn in the easiest way possible for them. Researchers have studied brain-processing patterns to detect the similarities or differences between how information is received and how the brain's right and left hemispheres act on it (Restak, 1979).

As an educator, being responsive to your students and understanding how their processing styles affect achievement is a necessity. The two major styles of gaining information are global and analytic.

Zenhausern (1980) linked students who have global learning-style preferences with students who process new information holistically. For global learners, it is crucial to understand an overall concept before focusing on details (Dunn, 1992). In addition, a holistic approach to instruction necessitates periodic relaxation breaks to decrease students' cognitive overload. In contrast, Zenhausern (1980) found that analytic learners use a left-processing style and learn backwards from global processors. He described the analytic student as using a sequential, step-by-step, building-block learning style and requiring facts to be taught in sequence to develop appropriate understanding. Freeley and Perrin (1987) refer to logical, analytical, and sequential learners as left-oriented, successive processors; they refer to holistic, intuitive, global learners as right-oriented simultaneous learners.

Global learners process information by looking at the whole picture and processing it simultaneously, interpreting it through their personal experiences and activities. An overview or summary facilitates comprehension by global learners. Information processing by analytic learners is detail-oriented; processing takes place step-by-step in a logical progression. Analytics like the picture divided into its component parts; outlines are helpful.

Information is absorbed differently by global and analytic learners. Globals tend to be more subjective, whereas analytics tend to be more objective. Conceptualization by globals occurs in a concrete manner as compared to by analytics who are relatively abstract.

Because globals are subjectively taking information in, they feel attached to it on a personal and real level. Analytics, on the other hand, are detached from personal involvement with information, which makes it relatively easy for them to recall rote items, such as multiplication tables.

GLOBAL AND ANALYTIC LEARNING-STYLE PREFERENCES

The Dunn and Dunn Learning-Style Model consists of five basic strands, including:

1. **Environmental** (needing sound versus quiet, low versus bright light, warm versus cool temperatures, and informal versus formal seating) while learning.

2. **Emotional** (high versus low motivation, persistence versus needing breaks, conformity versus nonconformity, and internal versus external needs for structure).

3. **Sociological** (learning alone, in a pair, with peers, in a small group, with an authoritative versus a collegial teacher, or in varied groupings).

4. **Physiological** (remembering new and difficult academic information most easily by hearing versus seeing versus manipulating versus experiencing, the time of day in which each person concentrates best, and individual needs for intake or mobility while learning).

5. **Psychological or cognitive** (global versus analytic processing).

Environmental Preferences

Many of the stimuli and elements of this model help educators adjust their lenses to see a clearer definition of what constitutes being global or analytic. In the environmental stimulus, sound significantly affects global processors; they prefer to have sound or music, television, and conversation while they study. In contrast, analytic processors prefer quiet while concentrating (Dunn, 1990, 1992; Dunn et al., 1990; Dunn, Cavanaugh, Eberle, & Zenhausern, 1982; Freeley & Perrin, 1987).

The amount of lighting required for these two processing types is different. Globals prefer soft, dim lighting when working on something new and difficult, whereas bright light works best for analytic processors (Dunn, 1990; Dunn et al., 1990; Dunn et al., 1982; Freeley & Perrin, 1987; Zenhausern, 1980). An informal seating arrangement is preferred by globals, whereas a traditional classroom of desks and chairs arranged in precise rows is fine for analytics (Dunn, 1990; Dunn et al., 1990; Freeley & Perrin, 1987; Zenhausern, 1980).

Emotional Preferences

Dunn (1990, 1992) reported that, in the emotional stimulus, persistence is usually representative of analytic processors who tend to complete one task before moving to another. Dunn and Dunn (1993) also reported that globals must be highly interested in what they are learning or they have little incentive to master the information. Frequent breaks, intake, and working on several projects simultaneously are what make globals' persistence levels low. Global processors reveal little persistence when working on only one task at a time. Instead, they work on several tasks simultaneously. This global trait also may be linked to a need to structure a task their way (Dunn, 1990).

Sociological Preferences

The sociological stimulus, including the elements of self, and/or working with an adult, were found to affect analytics infrequently. Dunn, Cavanaugh, Eberle, and Zenhausern (1982) reported that analytics tend to learn in different social patterns but that globals seem oriented toward working with peers when the material is difficult (Dunn et al., 1982; Freeley & Perrin, 1987).

Perceptual Preferences

Perceptually, whether students are auditory, tactile, kinesthetic, and/or visual plays an important role in how well they succeed. Teachers' lessons should complement a variety of perceptual strengths and their teaching strategies should address all perceptual elements, such as programmed learning sequences, contract activity packages, multisensory instructional packages, and creative assignments (Dunn & Dunn, 1993). Many globals and analytics often have strong tactual preferences and perform well with kinesthetic methods (Dunn et al., 1990; Dunn et al., 1982; Dunn & Dunn, 1993). In addition, intake is important to global processors; they often require snacking while learning something new and difficult (Dunn et al., 1990; Dunn et al., 1982).

Psychological Preferences

Hemisphericity is an element included in the Dunns' psychological stimulus. When students were taught according to their matched processing styles, significantly increased academic achievement was documented for both analytic and global learners (K–adult) (Brennan, 1984; Douglas, 1979; Dunn, 1990; Dunn et al., 1990; Jarsonbeck, 1984; Tanenbaum, 1982). Impulsive behavior was identified in both global and analytic processors, whereas reflective behavior only characterized analytic processors (Matson, 1980).

STRONGLY GLOBAL AND ANALYTIC PROCESSORS' LEARNING-STYLE CHARACTERISTICS AND RESPONSIVE CLASSROOM STRATEGIES

Dunn, Dunn, and Treffinger (1992) compared and contrasted the learning-style characteristics of strongly global and strongly analytic processors. They reported that strongly global processors preferred to have sound, soft lighting, informal seating, snacks, and several projects to do at the same time with frequent breaks. Those who are strongly analytic prefer a learning environment that includes quiet, bright illumination, a formal seating design, snacks after they have completed their task(s), and working on only one task at a time until it has been completed (Dunn, Dunn, & Treffinger, 1992). Figure 3.1 represents the link between processing and learning styles.

Once you know the learning-style preferences and information processing styles of your students, the challenge is to make the learning environment meet the needs of different types.

Conventional teaching methods respond to only one segment of the student population; therefore, it is imperative for teachers to adapt instruction to their students' styles. When teaching to globals, begin the lesson with a short, humorous (if possible) story related to the content, give an overall description of what will be taught, then focus on the details

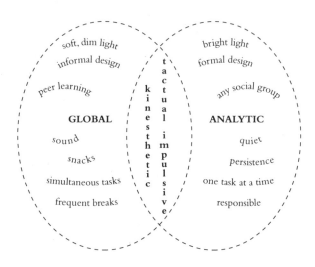

Figure 3.1 The Link between Processing and Learning Styles

and illustrate the text on the chalkboard with colors, pictures, and symbols. These strategies will also assist visual learners by:

- Addressing the social needs of the strongly global processor by allowing him or her to work with peers.
- Providing frequent breaks and snacks.
- Giving them choices in their assignments.
- Transforming your traditional classroom to one with a sense of informality.

Strongly analytic students, however, want you to begin the lesson with facts, provide an itemized list, and then a lesson summary leading them to understand the whole concept. Address each of the perceptual elements of their learning style; for visual learners, draw on the board or flip chart; for auditory learners, speak clearly and directly; for tactile learners, touch students' shoulders or wrists, encourage note taking or mapping, and teach them how to develop tactile resources; for kinesthetic learners (Dunn & Dunn, 1993), walk with the student or allow him or her to move in place while you are teaching.

Classroom Application

Applications to the classroom can be made easily with any of these strategies. Traditionally, nursing course assignments are "written in stone," with the instructor mandating format and procedure with no choice provided. Faculty members decide on their course assignments and how each is expected to be completed with strict adherence to their criteria. The content of one of my nursing courses was leadership and management of patient care.

During the spring semester, I administered the Productivity Environmental Preference Survey (PEPS) (Dunn, Dunn, & Price, 1986) to 35 baccalaureate nursing students enrolled in a senior year, second-semester nursing course. LaMothe et al. (1991, p. 30) described the PEPS as a "comprehensive learning style inventory for adults that measures a combination of elements that may influence student achievement and attitude." The content validity and reliability of the PEPS was established by assessing 433 baccalaureate-nursing students (LaMothe et al., 1991).

Students received an individual profile of their learning-style preferences. A group summary provided me with a composite of the entire class' learning-style preferences. After receiving the information, I distributed homework (study) prescriptions to each student. These prescriptions (study guides) were developed through the use of the *Homework Disc* software package used to analyze each student's preferred learning style based on his or her PEPS profiles (Dunn & Klavas, 1987). From the group summary obtained ($n = 35$), there were strong preferences for the following: auditory (17); learns best with peers (14); needs a warm temperature (19); needs structure (24); needs intake (22); works/learns best in afternoon (19); and requires mobility (14).

Contract Activity Packages

Dunn (1996, p. 43) suggests using contract activity packages (CAPs) as a "strategy to let motivated students progress at their own speed." A CAP consists of several components: (a) simply stated objective(s); (b) multisensory resource alternatives that teach the students the necessary information through their perceptual preferences; (c) activity alternatives in which students use the new information to create various instructional activities that foster their learning; (d) reporting alternatives that allow students various ways of presenting their newly discovered knowledge to their teacher and/or their peers; (e) the opportunity for students to work independently, in a pair, or with a group of peers; and (f) pretests, tests, and/or posttests to assess students' knowledge objectively. CAPs work well with students who are motivated, auditory, and nonconforming, as well as for those of varied academic levels who are either average, above-average, or gifted (Dunn, 1996; Dunn & Dunn, 1993).

On the basis of the learning-style profiles of my students, I decided to change the structure of the course assignments. I had prepared four required course assignments. Of these four, the Change Project and the Patient Care Delivery Models/Managed Care Project incorporated four to five activities students could choose to complete the assignment. Responses from my students were overwhelmingly positive. First they were surprised that they were allowed these opportunities; they had never experienced anything like this before in college. They loved that they could choose how to proceed with an assignment. Their grades were equally positive. They reflected critical thinking skills, quality written work, and creativity. Since students had received individual PEPS printouts and their homework prescriptions, they knew who wanted to work alone and they were allowed to do so. For those whose learning style was either in a pair or with peers, they too were afforded the opportunity to learn and complete their assignments in their own style. Some students, although very few (3 of 35), had no preferences.

SUMMARY

Research indicates that individuals have diverse methods of processing information, ranging on a continuum from highly analytic to highly global. These two opposite processing styles are related to other learning-style preferences, including sound, light, design, intake, and mobility. When students are taught with interventions that are congruent with their cognitive processing style, significant increases in academic achievement result.

Nurse educators need to apply this research by assessing students' information-processing styles, implementing classroom interventions that accommodate a variety of different styles, and providing opportunities for students to learn independently in ways that complement their learning-style strengths.

Chapter 4

Teaching Health Information Management Students through Their Individual Learning Styles

Rose Frances Lefkowitz, MPA, RRA

Stimuli   ELEMENTS

Environmental

Emotional

Sociological

Physiological

Psychological

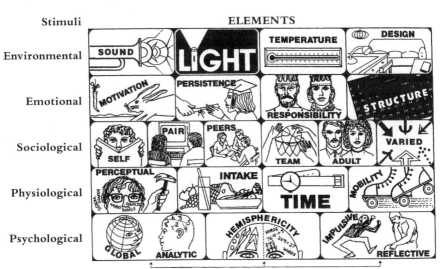

Simultaneous or Successive Processing

How do you teach your health information management students? Do you stand in front of a lectern to speak and compel your students to listen for 2 hours—or more? Do you prefer to show videotapes, slides, and/or transparencies, so that your students see what you are attempting to teach? Is your preference taking students to the microcomputer laboratory to participate in a hands-on approach to learning? Does your presentation include any kinesthetic activities, such as a walking tour into the world of health records and health information management? You are teaching, but are you certain that your students are learning?

If you teach, you have a teaching style. Have you considered the possibility that your students' learning styles may not be compatible with your teaching style? Learning style is the ". . . way students begin to concentrate, process, and retain new and difficult information" (Dunn & Dunn, 1993, p. 2). During the past decade, students' learning styles have made gradual and exciting differences in the way *I* teach my students.

I am an assistant professor and senior faculty member who has been teaching basic and advanced courses in health information management for approximately 15 years. For many years, my approach to teaching was clearly traditional—I lectured; my students listened. When some students grasped the information immediately, whereas others had difficulty understanding and retaining what I presented, I assumed that the two groups were opposite ends of a continuum—one was motivated, the other was not; one had studied, the other had not; one was bright, the other had been admitted erroneously.

During the early 1990s, my teaching began to change. One of my colleagues, an assistant professor of diagnostic medical imaging, asked if she could discuss the concept of learning styles with students in one of my classes and invite them to participate in an experimental project in which she was interested. Listening to her presentation, I realized that there are many approaches to teaching content. What appeared to be crucial was that whichever method I used needed to accommodate the learning style of each student.

Over the past six years, I have become convinced that identifying my students' learning styles and then presenting information in responsive ways is worth the effort and time. The results—improved student academic achievement and attitudes toward learning—make my task worthwhile.

ANALYTIC VERSUS GLOBAL LEARNERS

Students are told at the very beginning of the program that each has a unique style of learning new and difficult information. No style is better or worse than another. Most students process information in one of two different ways—analytically or globally, although some use both styles some of the time. Analytical learners prefer a step-by-step, sequential explanation that gradually builds to an understanding of the topic or concept being taught. Global learners prefer to process new and difficult information holistically; they need to understand how the topic or concept relates to them and their lives before they can concentrate on the details and facts. Global learners need to see how the topic or concept affects them personally before they are willing to invest effort in studying. According to Dunn & Dunn, (1993), approximately 55 percent of the adult population is global and 28 percent is analytic. The remaining adults process information based on their reactions to the situation. The following attributes tend to be characteristic of analytic versus global learners when studying challenging academic material:

- **Analytics** need quiet without interruptions; they like bright lighting, formal desk-and-chair seating designs, no intake, and working on a task until it has been completed.

- **Globals** need sound (music or conversation), many short breaks, soft lighting, an informal lounge chair, carpeting, a sofa, intake, and working on several tasks simultaneously.

TEXTBOOKS OF HEALTH INFORMATION MANAGEMENT

The textbooks used to study health information management all seem to have been written by analytics; understandably they are best understood by analytics. The most recognized textbook of this discipline is *Health Information Management* (Huffman, 1994). A significant amount of material of the certification board questions is referenced or drawn from this textbook. I wrote my chapter in this text analytically—just as I used to teach in the classroom—one analytic presenting facts and details to another. I had not realized that I was losing the global students merely because of the way the information was presented to them. I was determined to change the methods I used; capturing my global students became top priority. Gradually, my teaching adapted to the type of learners in each class. I began by introducing the Dunn and Dunn Learning-Styles Model to assess the learning styles of my students.

DUNN AND DUNN LEARNING-STYLES MODEL

The figure that opens this chapter provides an overview of the Dunn and Dunn model, which consists of five basic strands (inclusive of 21 distinct learning-style elements in all):

1. **Environmental** (needing sound versus quiet, low versus bright light, warm versus cool temperatures, and informal versus formal seating) while learning.

2. **Emotional** (high versus low motivation, persistence versus needing breaks, conformity versus nonconformity, and internal versus external needs for structure.

3. **Sociological** (learning alone, in a pair, with peers, in a small group, with an authoritative versus a collegial teacher, or in varied groupings.

4. **Physiological** (remembering new and difficult academic information most easily by hearing versus seeing versus manipulating versus experiencing; the time of day in which each person concentrates best, and individual needs for intake or mobility while learning).

5. **Psychological** (global versus analytic processing).

Learning-Style Assessments of Students

All incoming junior students are required to take Health Information Management I, a fundamental and comprehensive overview course. These students are followed for a 2-year journey through their experiences at college. After a brief presentation on background and supporting research, students in this course volunteered to take the Productivity Environmental Preference Survey (PEPS) (Dunn, Dunn, & Price, 1982, 1989) to identify their individual learning styles.

The PEPS consists of 100 dichotomous questions that elicit self-diagnostic responses relating to the Dunn and Dunn model, comprising 21 distinct learning style elements on a 5-point Likert scale (Nelson et al., 1993). This survey is one of the few instruments with good reliability and validity (Griggs, Griggs, Dunn, & Ingham, 1994). Within the past decade, the following studies have indicated predictive validity of the PEPS (Buell & Buell, 1987; Dunn, Bruno, et al., 1990; Ingham, 1991; LaMothe et al., 1991; Lenehan, Dunn, Ingham, Murray, & Signer, 1994).

Students were given individualized learning-style data, and an individual counseling session was held to explain the meaning of the results. A written interpretation of the results, based on each student's learning-style profile, was translated into an individual prescription generated by the Homework Disc (Dunn & Klavas, 1990). Diagnosis and homework prescription was instrumental in making their interests in learning come alive again. Frequently heard comments included: "Until now, no professor ever cared about the way that I learned" and "I am going to enjoy studying this topic because you're taking such an interest in how I learn." Following up on the results, a review of a PEPS group summary gave me the information I needed to present the course information in a variety of different ways. Each student had different perceptual strengths: some preferred to hear information (auditory); others wanted to see it (visual); some preferred hands-on learning (tactual); others wanted to experience the information (kinesthetic). Most students can learn new and difficult information when it is presented through their primary perceptual strength and then reinforced through their secondary perceptual strength to ensure long-term retention of information.

Development of Instructional Resources

I now know who is global and who is analytic. I know the primary, secondary, and perhaps even the tertiary perceptual strengths of my students. I can vary my teaching presentations accordingly by supplementing my lectures with auditory, visual, tactual, and kinesthetic resources according to perceptual strength preferences, or by supplementing these resources with my lectures. What do I do with the analytic textbook that comprises a most significant portion of the certification board questions on the national examination? Develop instructional resources to complement the learning styles of the student. The PEPS group summary indicated that the students have a visual and/or tactual strength. All students tested were motivated and/or in need of structure.

This chapter highlights one type of resource developed by health information management students: the programmed learning sequence (PLS). Based on the Dunn and Dunn Learning-Style Model, the PLS is designed to structure learning for those with visual strength. It also is useful to students who are motivated and tactual. The PLS can be used for studying in pairs or independently. It may be used in a classroom library, corridor, or in an instructional resource center as well as at home, because it accommodates each student's environmental and physical preferences (Dunn & Dunn, 1993, p. 203). It is excellent for students who prefer direction (structure).

One semester all students received a course outline for Health Information Management I, which required that they develop a PLS for one of the chapters of the text *Health Information Management* (Huffman, 1994). The intent behind this requirement was that they would read the chapter assigned thoroughly and *know* the information presented. Thus, students would develop a PLS to ultimately help current and future classmates learn new and difficult health information management concepts. The PLS is comprised of a story related to the topic focus to appeal to the global learner and explain the topic prior to presenting facts. It then includes a structured presentation of information contained within the chapter frame by frame. Review and mastery of the information may be presented any number of ways. Quite often material is presented in the form of a word search, crossword puzzle, matching definitions related to key concepts, or a series of questions to be answered. Included in the PLS are tactual (hands-on manipulatives) responsive to students who prefer that modality. Such tactual resources may include construction of a puzzle in the form of a related topic or a unique mini-electroboard which lights up at the touch of a correct response. Only one item is presented at a time; students become active learners and are informed immediately as to the correctness of the response. Students may not continue to the next frame (page) until each previous frame has been completed and understood (Dunn & Dunn, 1993, p. 206). PLS topics developed for this course include both an analytic title and a global title to appeal to both types of learners. Some sample PLS topics developed by the health information management students are listed below:

- Legal Aspects of Medical Records Information: Witness to the Crime!

- International Classification of Diseases: Coding Counts! (9th Revision (ICD-9-CM))

- Content of the Mental Health Patient's Record: Use Your Head!

- Nomenclatures and Classification Systems: World of Codes: Simply about Complex

- Management of Health Information Department Personnel: Don't Get Personal with Personnel

The following 25 characteristics are essential to the development of a PLS (Dunn & Dunn, 1993, pp. 269–270):

1. An attractive cover in a shape related to content.

2. Both an analytic and a global title (humor, play on words).

3. Clearly stated objectives.

4. Specific directions for the student to follow.

5. A global beginning.

6. When possible, the story woven through the entire PLS.

7. Interesting upbeat phrases rather than academic directives.

8. Step-by-step sequencing.

9. Actual teaching with the identical concept or material repeated in different ways on several frames.

10. Answers on the back of the frame, accompanied by humor, jokes, and illustrations.

11. Illustrations related to the text, in color.

12. Varied questioning types.

13. An accompanying tape.

14. Answers provided in complete statements.

15. No "yes" or "no" answers.

16. An interdisciplinary theme for global students.

17. Appropriate review frames.

18. Built-in tactual reviews.

19. Neatness, attractiveness, legibility.

20. Correct spelling and grammar.

21. Original and creative touches.

22. Themes or ideas related to students' interests, lifestyles, or talents.

23. A choice or two, at times.

24. Laminated easy-to-handle frames.

25. Frames that will turn in the correct position (not upside-down).

Students who can benefit from using this instructional resource are encouraged to take the PLS home, to the library, to the classroom, or wherever to learn new and difficult information on health information management. An audiotape accompanies this resource for those who have an auditory strength. Each student developed a PLS on a certain chapter/topic and later exchanged PLS for review of other chapters/topics to master the material. As a result of incorporating this instructional resource, as well as learning-style theory into the course, students increased their scores on examinations based upon the material learned through the development of the PLS. Further, students enjoyed developing the materials and displayed a more favorable outlook toward learning.

CONCLUSION

The juniors are now seniors and almost ready to graduate. The knowledge they have gained will be lasting. Examination scores and attitudes indicate that a definite increase has occurred. The ultimate test of long-term retention and successful academic achievement will be the results of the national certification board examination.

Chapter 5

Teaching Baccalaureate Diagnostic Medical Sonography Students with a Learning-Style Approach

Joyce A. Miller, EdD, MM, RDMS

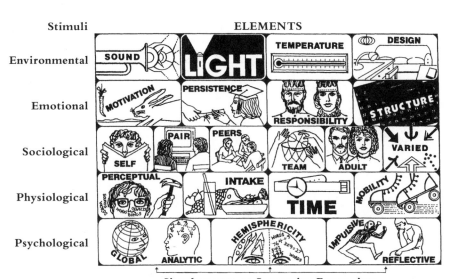

Stimuli   ELEMENTS

Environmental

Emotional

Sociological

Physiological

Psychological

Simultaneous or Successive Processing

From college students' perspectives, as Claxton and Murrell (1987) reported, knowledge of their learning styles improved course performance. The next year, Anderson (1988) urged examination of the relationships among students' (a) knowledge of their learning styles, (b) academic achievement, (c) use of congruent study strategies while learning, and (d) rates of retention. It was reasonable to suggest instruction based on individuals' learning styles for unsuccessful students, but it is unlikely that Claxton, Murrel, or Anderson would have perceived a need for learning style-responsive approaches with the able students in our highly competitive college of health-related professions! I doubt that many researchers could have anticipated the improved test scores that resulted from capitalizing on the learning styles of the achievers in our traditional program.

In 1970, the State University of New York Health Science Center at Brooklyn initiated the first baccalaureate degree program in diagnostic medical sonography (ultrasound). Because it was the first of its kind in the United States, our curriculum and instruction followed the typical medical model—professorial lectures, examination of slides in class, and the scanning of patients at a clinical site. Because we were perceived as an innovative program, faculty conscientiously sought to reflect conservative pedagogy.

However, two decades later in 1990, the construct of learning style, as defined by the Dunn and Dunn Model, began to make some subtle, exciting, and profound changes in staff philosophy and curriculum. This chapter explains how learning-style theory practices were operationalized in our ultrasound program.

STEP 1: BECOMING AWARE OF LEARNING STYLES

Dunn and Dunn (1993) describe learning style as ". . . the way in which individuals begin to concentrate on, process, internalize, and retain new

Table 5.1   The Dunn and Dunn Learning-Styles Model: Productivity Environmental Preference Survey Elements

Environmental Elements

1.	Noise level	Silence versus sound
2.	Light	Dim versus bright light
3.	Temperature	Cool versus warm temperature
4.	Design	Informal versus formal setting

Emotional Elements

5.	Motivation	Self-motivated
6.	Persistence	Persistence versus periodic breaks
7.	Responsibility	Conformity versus nonconformity
8.	Structure	Internal versus external structure

Sociological Elements

9.	Alone/Peer	Learning alone versus peer-oriented learner
10.	Authority figures	Authority figures absent-present; requiring versus not requiring feedback
11.	Learns in several ways	Requiring patterns and routines versus variety

Physiological Elements

12.	Auditory	Remembers ¾ of what is heard
13.	Visual	Remembers ¾ of what is read/seen
14.	Tactile	Remembers ¾ of what is written/manipulated
15.	Kinesthetic	Remembers ¾ of what is experienced
16.	Intake	Learns best while eating/drinking
17.	Evening-morning	Evening versus morning alert
18.	Late morning	Functions best in late morning
19.	Afternoon	Functions best in afternoon
20.	Mobility	Learning while passive versus mobile

and difficult information" (p. 2). They perceive of 20 different variables that may or may not affect each individual differentially on a continuum that indicates each person's strengths. (See the figure on the first page of the chapter and Table 5.1.) These strengths either inhibit or complement an individual's ability to perform.

The Dunns' definition of learning style increasingly intruded on my concentration as I lectured each day in, what I perceived to be, a scholarly and erudite manner. Without fail, certain students entered into what appeared to be a semicomatose trance. They periodically struggled to keep their eyes open and their heads erect. On occasion, some closed their eyes, leaned their chins or heads on their hands, squirmed and wriggled in their seats, and appeared—in the most euphemistic of catch phrases—to be "out of it."

These student behaviors are not unknown to college professors, but two interesting things invariably occurred. While this first group struggled to maintain erect bodies, other students simultaneously moved to the edge of their seats and seemed totally absorbed in every word I uttered. After reading about learning styles, my seemingly bored students' decorum suggested that it might not have been my presentation that was losing the group with the diminishing attention span; conceivably, it could have been the dissonance between their learning style and my teaching style, which reduced my responsibility and placed the cause directly on the mismatch. After all, my lectures obviously interested the group straining to hear my every word!

STEP 2: BECOMING AWARE OF THE LEARNING STYLES OF HIGH-ACHIEVERS

Researchers have consistently reported that the learning-styles of high achievers were significantly different from those of students who did not perform well in school (Griggs & Dunn, 1984). The gifted invariably were persistant (Dunn & Price, 1980; Griggs & Price, 1980; Price, Dunn,

Dunn, & Griggs, 1981; Ricca, 1983), highly motivated (Cody, 1983; Cross, 1982; Dunn & Price, 1980; Griggs & Price, 1980; Price et al., 1981), and preferred learning alone rather than with others (Cross, 1982; Griggs & Price, 1980; Kreitner, 1981; Price et al., 1981; Ricca, 1983)— unless those "others" were similarly achieving gifted peers (Perrin, 1984).

Many high IQ students required extreme quiet (Cody, 1983) and bright light (Griggs & Price, 1980) when concentrating on demanding academic tasks. Moreover, in contrast with average and low achievers, gifted students often resisted learning directly from their teachers, which is what my class lectures had required.

Dunn and Price (1980) reported that many gifted students preferred little structure while learning; they wanted to do thing *their* way rather than by following directions. A preference for low, rather than high structure, was another element that discriminated between high and low achievers. Indeed, students with an IQ between 120 and 130, in the 90th percentile or above in reading or mathematics, were often extremely independent (Stewart, 1981; Wasson, 1980), internally controlled, and desirous of providing their own structure (Cross, 1982; Dunn & Price, 1980; Kreitner, 1981; Ricca, 1983; Stewart, 1981).

High-achieving students remember three quarters of what they learn by listening. They also learn visually (by seeing or reading), tactually (by handling materials, note taking, or manipulating items), and kinesthetically (by active involvement and experiencing). In contrast, average and underachieving students usually learn well through one modality only— often the tactual or kinesthetic. Although gifted students *can* learn by listening to lectures or tapes, several different diagnostic instruments and extensive interviews document that high achievers strongly dislike recitation, lectures, class discussions, and drill (Ricca, 1983). Indeed, Wasson (1980) reported that gifted students preferred learning with games, projects (kinesthetic), independent studies, and Programmed Learning Sequences. Peer teaching ranked fourth in Ricca's (1983) findings and was preferred only by gifted students permitted to learn with equally gifted classmates (Perrin, 1984).

STEP 3: COUNSELING

I introduced my students to learning style by explaining its meaning and the variables that comprise the Dunns' model. The juniors and seniors were so interested that I also described some of the research that supported the model. They were intrigued, easily absorbed the construct, and volunteered to take a learning-style assessment to identify their styles.

I tested each class with the Productivity Environmental Preference Survey (PEPS) (Dunn, Dunn, & Price, 1982, 1989) and, when the results were returned, offered each student an individual counseling session to explain the results. At first, I personally interpreted each profile, but quickly learned to use St. John's University's Homework Disc, a computer software package that both interprets individuals' PEPS profiles and prescribes guidelines for studying based on each person's learning style strengths (Dunn & Klavas, 1990). Students were receptive to and grateful for these analyses. Whereas some had been aware of their learning styles before the counseling session, many had no understanding of how to capitalize on their styles. From the analysis of their strengths, all were able to concretize study options effective for them.

The most striking reaction was from one student who had many elements that comprise a global processing style. Maria had tested low in both the auditory and visual modalities, but expressed strong preferences for tactual and kinesthetic learning. She had been one of the students who consistently struggled to remain attentive, often leaving for breaks after 10 minutes of lecture.

Maria confided that she had always felt "different" from and inferior to other students in the class; she had only "just managed to get through" some courses. When assured that her learning style was acceptable and counseled on how to capitalize on her tactual and kinesthetic strengths, both her attitude and achievement improved considerably. Assessing for learning styles and then counseling incoming juniors has now become an established procedure in our program.

Having intelligent, highly achieving diagnostic medical sonography students in my classes had lulled me into thinking that each should be alert and responsive during lectures. Interpretation of my students' PEPS printouts alerted me to the fact that many of those young adults did not have a typical achiever's profile. Most were persistent and motivated, needed quiet, and preferred learning alone, but some preferred learning with an authority figure and, invariably, these were the students who intently listened to my every word.

In one class, I had a sizeable group that was far more tactual and kinesthetic than auditory. After I gave them guidelines for studying based on their tactual or kinesthetic strengths, most reported relative ease of learning and remembering the information.

STEP 4: APPLYING LEARNING STYLES TO TEACHING

I began modifying my presentations by beginning lessons tactually—with physical examinations of anatomic models prior to discussion. I placed some key questions on the board and provided for their sociological differences by permitting students to work alone, in pairs, with a small group, or by sitting near me. I encouraged them to handle the equipment probes and to perform some ultrasound scanning with the help of volunteer students in the lab. I then followed up with a lecture and slide presentation on the topic, reinforcing information the students had been exposed to tactually and kinesthetically (by doing). It was immediately apparent that students were actively involved more than ever. Furthermore, none seemed bored during the lecture, which was provided during the latter part of each lesson. Students began volunteering and enthusiastically answered the questions I posed! The differences between their posture and contributions during this learning-style lesson and my traditional lectures were immediately apparent—and continued all semester!

STEP 5: DEVELOPING INSTRUCTIONAL RESOURCES

I was intrigued that the research on gifted students' learning styles reflects so closely many of the traits revealed on my students' PEPS profiles. Many of my students were persistent, motivated, preferred to learn kinesthetically or tactually, and in a quiet environment. A few were authority-oriented, but most enjoyed working independently without much external structure. Many actually disliked lectures, recitations, and drill and preferred programmed learning sequences (PLS) (Dunn & Dunn, 1993). The latter was an approach I had not used, but when I researched the technique, I found that PLSs incorporated global anecdotal beginnings, illustrations and humor, visual and tactual cues, and periodic games for tactual reinforcements (Dunn & Dunn, 1993). I decided to try one or two.

I developed a few PLSs and integrated them into my course curricula. I doubted that my relatively sophisticated, young adult high-achievers would appreciate them. On the other hand, the PLSs *did* respond to many of my students' learning-style traits.

PLSs are designed to present new and difficult information in small, discrete steps that promote learning without direct supervision by an instructor. They are appropriate for students who enjoy some structure while learning in a quiet environment, have good visual or tactual strengths, prefer to learn individually or in a pair, and are motivated and persistent (Dunn & Dunn, 1993). Many of my students fit that profile.

I developed two PLSs for my ultrasound class: one in a book format and the other on multimedia software for the computer. Several research studies have demonstrated that computer-assisted instruction is versatile and can accommodate various learning styles (Bratt & Vockell, 1986; Khoiny, 1995; Koch, Rankin, & Stewart, 1990). I wanted to compare the effects of learning traditionally, lectures and accompanying visuals with illustrations, with learning from a booktype PLS as described by Dunn and Dunn (1993). I also wanted to compare the effects of these two methods with those of a computer PLS.

My first PLS topic on normal renal ultrasound was titled "Joe Montana Learns All about Passing—A Kidney Stone That Is!" In a humorous vein, the text described the anatomy of Montana's kidneys and the protocols for performing a sonogram of a normal kidney. I included diagrams, sonograms, and lots of jokes. After each frame (page) of material, the students were questioned about the information that appeared on it, and then received immediate feedback from answers provided on the following frame.

The multimedia interactive PLS titled "A Saga of Footballs and Kidneys" was a sequel that probed the complex topic of renal pathology. It involved critical thinking skills concerned with knowledge of anatomy and pathophysiology of the disease processes. Students then learned how to relate this information to patient history. Students had to synthesize this knowledge with how pathology is manifested on a sonogram.

This PLS began with Joe Montana being "pink-footballed" from his team, falling into a dream state, and being scanned for renal pathology by Sophie, the Sonographer. I developed this resource using Multimedia Toolbook 3.0 by Assymetrix, a Windows-authoring software package that creates multiple-screen applications with pages in a book. More than 20 sonograms depicting various pathologies were scanned into the program, which also included graphics, diagrams, freehand cartoons, puns, and rhymes.

For my cross-sectional anatomy course, I developed a book-format PLS titled "Axial Anatomy of the Brain: Sam the Sonographer Sneaks a Snack at a Smorgasbord." As in the previous resources, it began with a humorous introduction. Contained in the text was the detailed anatomy of the brain using computerized tomography scans, diagrams, charts, cartoons, and jokes. Information was mastered by reading the text and accompanying illustrations, answering the questions at the bottom of each frame, and seeing the immediate feedback and the additional humor where appropriate.

Who would have ever anticipated college students loving to learn new and difficult material? My students so enjoyed these resources that they quickly learned the material, obtained excellent test scores and pleaded for more. There were no more, and that is why I challenged these formerly somnanbulant souls to develop their own.

STEP 6: STUDENT CONSTRUCTION OF LEARNING-STYLE RESOURCES

Some of our graduates aspire to becoming ultrasound college professors; and for that reason, our program includes a team-taught teaching methods course that includes alternative instructional systems. In one of the course modules, I introduced the PLS and several other innovative resources: Contract Activity Packages (CAPs), Multisensory Instructional Packages (MIPS) (Dunn & Dunn, 1993). I provided a short "how to" introduction, showed samples of each resource, and made available easy-to-read descriptive articles and the Dunns' book (1993) to provide guidelines for resource development.

STEP 7: APPLICATIONS TO OUR CURRICULUM COURSE WORK

We then assigned the task of constructing these materials for the topics related to our curriculum and permitted the students to work alone, in pairs, or in a team. Many chose to work together in teams, but several chose to work independently.

The results of the assignments were astonishing. PLSs on heart disease, placentation, congenital birth defects, gallbladder pathology, and maternal diabetes were designed that covered the topics thoroughly and in an interesting and most arresting manner! Two students swore they spent over 100 hours developing a sophisticated computer PLS on the brain—and the completed product made the claim credible. An MIP on the embryology of the heart was sensational, and the student who developed it donated it to our program after he graduated.

We obtained permission to duplicate original resources to be used as alternative learning resources for future students in our program. Faculty were delighted with the students' enthusiasm and projects. We look forward to making these instructional resources available to those students who will need different ways of learning the required content next year. We will give the identical assignment to our classes next year and hope to gradually develop a library of innovative resources to teach in our curriculum.

Our students have acquired both knowledge and the experience of alternative teaching practices—information that will help them teach themselves and others whose learning styles are either nontraditional or require instructional variety.

STEP 8: REDESIGNING THE COLLEGE INSTRUCTIONAL ENVIRONMENT

Learning style has made faculty aware of how important sound, light, temperature, seating, snacking, and mobility can be to some learners. With new insight, we examined our lab, long considered a boon to ultrasound teaching and a source of great faculty pride. The lab included several ultrasound machines to permit extensive student practice, several stretchers, a lucite cadaver divided into axial sections for the study of cross-sectional anatomy, a variety of anatomic models, sonogram viewing screens, a television and videocassette recorder, a carousel slide projector, tables, and other items.

With an eye toward creating alternative areas to provide comfort for different types of learners, we reorganized the equipment and resources to provide separate sections where students could sit at formal, library tables and chairs, and an informal section that included a donated couch. We also permitted snacking, but the rules for cleaning up and maintaining the environment were clearly stated. One corner of the lab was established as a media center. It included the television and slide projector for those who wanted to use them. A scanning area was established near the ultrasound machines to allow students to scan each other; a partition was ordered to allow privacy for students needing to partially disrobe. The lighting in the lab can be adjusted and adapted to different tasks.

RESULTS

Beyond this anecdotal report, when I examined the comparative results of the three instructional strategies (traditional versus book-PLS versus computer PLS) (Miller, 1997), results indicated that my students had earned significantly higher achievement and attitude test scores with the book-PLS than with either the traditional lecture or the multimedia package. Interestingly, the few students who had scored better through my lectures were the *only* ones in my classes who were identified as highly authority oriented by the PEPS. They, therefore, preferred learning with an authoritative figure present—me! Students who scored better with the book-PLS than with the computer-PLS had a strong need for learning in a quiet, informal environment.

In general, almost all students performed better with the PLSs than with my lectures. However, fewer students scored better with the computer-PLS than with the book-PLS, which they were permitted to work with it anywhere. Thus, students could settle into an area that was acoustically comfortable and with the seating and illumination each preferred. Interestingly, students whose PEPS profiles indicated a need for intake while concentrating, performed better in this classroom environment where they could snack as they worked than in the computer lab where food and drinks were not permitted.

SUMMARY

For almost three decades, the major tenet of our program has been to graduate diagnostic medical sonographers who excel in both didactic knowledge and clinical experience. Several learning-style approaches have helped us reach that goal. We recommend any or all of the following for health professionals who teach:

1. Identify students' learning styles and make them aware of their strengths.

2. Distribute homework prescriptions that show students how to study through their strongest learning-style traits.

3. Redesign the instructional environment (classrooms, labs, study areas) to provide for as many learning-style differences as feasible in your situation. You don't have to do everything; however, everything you do will help.

4. Develop at least one PLS to teach on a curriculum topic. Try it with your students, see how many enjoy learning with it, and determine how well they achieve when using it.

5. Require that students create PLSs on a different topic of your curriculum. Share those with other students and keep them for use by subsequent classes.

6. Repeat the processes described in 4 and 5 with a CAP or MIP. As you move through this process, note the relative gains of students and their attitudes toward learning. You will be impressed with their enthusiasm and interest.

7. Consider the PLSs, CAPS, and MIPS that are available as alternative approaches to teaching curriculum content. Encourage students to experiment with them and to create their own.

8. Become acquainted with other approaches the Dunns (1993) advocate. Everything we've tried has worked well with some students; overall, my colleagues, students, and I have been very pleased with the results.

Chapter 6

Learning Styles-Based Instruction: Eleven Steps over the Brick Wall

Lauren E. O'Hare, MSN, RN

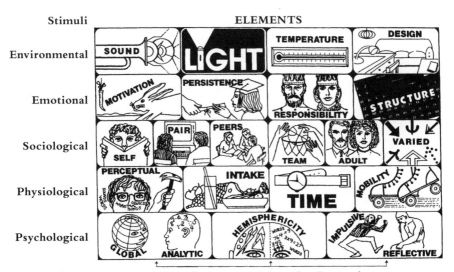

If you are reading this chapter, feel a bit queasy and say, "It won't work at the college level," you're reacting exactly as I did the first time I heard about learning styles. I intuitively knew it was exactly what many elementary and some secondary students would thrive on, but there was no way I could imagine teaching the young adults in my nursing and health classes using different variations of acoustics, illumination, temperature, and seating designs.

The first time I voiced my recalcitrance to my professor, I hit a brick wall. She smiled as she softly said, "You need to try it, or you can't pass this course." "This course" was the first in a long doctoral sequence, and this woman was one of the core professors. What choice did I have?

I teach baccalaureate nursing at a private college of approximately 2,300 students. My students are bright. They vary in motivational levels, but most are industrious young adults who want very much to succeed. The course work is challenging, and there are many standardized tests to be passed along the way. How on earth would I be able to teach in different ways to students with different learning styles and still maintain our nursing curriculum standards that would someday lead to state licensing?

STEP 1: MAKING INSTRUCTIONAL RESOURCES

I followed the directions for completing one contract activity package (CAP) (Dunn & Dunn, 1993) on a required curriculum unit, the heart. CAPs are designed for motivated, auditory/visual, fairly independent students who may need either structure or options, as their learning-style profile indicates. The basic CAP included clearly stated objectives, alternative resources, an option of creative activities in which students could demonstrate their mastery of the unit's objectives, ways in which the original activities might be shared with classmates, at least three small-group strategies for the very difficult objectives, and a test. I assumed that at least some of my students could handle this instructional resource.

The part of the CAP that troubled me was the resource alternatives. These allow students to choose the materials with which they learn the required CAP's objectives, and the materials include everything from classroom tapes students can make of my lectures to assignments I require them to read, to whatever they can find on the topic in the library, such as videotapes, transparencies, or models. However, CAPs also require tactual manipulatives, such as flip chutes, electroboards, pic-a-holes, and multipart task cards—elementary-school devices in which students read questions related to the objectives and either piece together answers or use manipulatives to find hints. CAPs also require a large piece of plastic to be place on the floor. Students choose questions in this activity and find matching answers that teach the unit's objectives by physically moving from one spot on the plastic to another—somewhat like the game Twister. Whereas the CAP itself hadn't caused too much stress because it resembled something like an independent study I had experienced during one of my graduate classes, the tactual and kinesthetic plastic floor game caused me real concern.

STEP 2: INTRODUCING THE RESOURCES TO COLLEGE STUDENTS

I struggled for weeks with the decision to introduce the tactual and kinesthetic materials. After all, this nursing course was a core, adult health course that focused heavily on assignments, diagnosis, treatment, and evaluation of multiple disease processes. I had doubts that these young adults, ranging in age from 18 to 45, would ever be receptive to this type of teaching. They were paying a good amount for tuition and the last thing I wanted to hear was, "I'm paying X amount of dollars to play games in class? My parents/spouse/loan officer will complain!" I even questioned my own motivation to remain in that doctoral program. Did I really need the degree?

Then reason overcame hysteria. I thought, "What do I have to lose?" There was a tremendous amount of research on learning styles that consistently reported statistically increased achievement and attitude test scores whenever this model had been introduced to college students. If it failed, I could show the professor that it wasn't for lack of effort that it hadn't worked with my nursing students. If I were in this program to learn, shouldn't I at least try? What if this brick-wall-of-a-professor was correct, and it really did work? What kind of teacher would I be if I refused to try?

At every session of that semester, we were required to read one experimental study after the next. Each study appeared to consistently support the fact that students are different from each other and that what works with one is not necessarily effective with another. The teaching that helps one student succeed may actually prevent another student from learning. Wasn't I being inflexible to refuse to even see what would happen? In addition, classmates in the same course who also taught at local colleges, were reporting almost weekly successes. And every time one of them described how their students had become exhilarated over learning-style resources, the professor slyly glanced my way.

STEP 3: THE DAY OF RECKONING

What finally made me sufficiently courageous to try the material was that I knew it was my responsibility to present that complex unit on the heart to the class. I also had to prepare them to take the state licensing examination within one year. I realized it would be unfair to hold back the information on the heart and that identifying their learning styles might possibly teach these students to capitalize on their strengths. How could I not even try?

As my panic slowly dissipated, I decided that it would be no holds barred. I began by explaining the concept of learning style to the class and reporting just a little of the research—which I was beginning to know by heart. My students became genuinely interested in learning about themselves, and as each learning-style element was described, they began picturing themselves in various studying situations. Their heads nodded in agreement, many exclaimed, "That's me!" and others offered anecdotes about what they had actually done to accommodate some aspects of their style. Others expressed curiosity and asked if I could test them to reveal what their "style strengths" were. Many were eager for more information.

Then I unveiled the floor game to teach the basic objectives of the unit on the heart. To my surprise, the students' first reaction was *shock* to see how creative I had been! They also were pleased that I had cared enough about them to do "all that extra work." (Their comments made me wonder what they had thought of my teaching to that point!) They then prodded me to show them how to learn with the game and, almost as they began gathering the information, they voiced pleasure—without prompting: "We like it! What a fun way to learn!" They seemed happy to be released from the typical lecture/video/transparency methods I had been using, and they thoroughly enjoyed learning through active involvement rather than in their seats! Instead of chaos, however, they behaved exuberantly, bur orderly, and took turns, helped each other, formed competitive teams to see which group could master the most information during the period, and appeared to be genuinely enjoying the new method.

STEP 4: STUDENTS' REACTIONS TO THE INSTRUCTIONAL RESOURCES

Being able to mobilize themselves and experiment with a new resource was appealing to many. A few had difficulty playing the game on the floor and, instead, attached it to the wall. Some liked the change; others could not quite adapt to the movement it required and questioned whether this was the only new way I had to teach them. That was my golden opportunity! I realized that I now had the perfect moment for showing them another learning-style resource.

I introduced the CAP to the class and encouraged those who wanted to work with this structured outline to choose the resources with which they could master the objectives on the heart and proceed on their own. A few found the CAP enticing; others said it "looked too hard." I showed the remaining students a programmed learning sequence (PLS)— another learning-style resource that introduced the heart through an anecdotal story relating the content directly to them and their lives. The PLS included the identical objectives as the CAP, but it taught in a much more structured manner, provided no options, included small amounts of information on each frame, followed with questions and immediate feedback answers, interspersed the answers with jokes, teasing, and illustrations, and periodically inserted tactual, gamelike reinforcements of the material that had already been introduced. I can't tell you how anxious the students were to get their hands on the PLS! They read either independently, in pairs, or in groups. They laughed at the humor and responded accordingly. They began to recognize that the PLS was teaching exactly the same objectives as the CAP and the floor game, and gradually they realized how much they already had learned in just the first 10 to 15 minutes with the floor game!

Students were excited and focused only on obtaining answers to the questions related to the objectives. Within 15 minutes, some tired of the floor game and moved into the group using the PLS. Others wanted to know what else I had created to teach about the heart. I displayed the tactuals—the electroboard that lit up when the correct question and answer were joined by the two "arms" of a continuity tester; the task cards in which one half of a heart with a question related to the objectives could be matched correctly with the other half of the heart with the correct answer; the flip chute in which a question was deposited into a box and, as if by magic, the correct answer popped out! These adults, whom I had feared would be exasperated by the gamelike resources, became entranced. As soon as they realized that each resource taught exactly the same information—although lots of it, they formed groups to see which team could learn most in the shortest amount of time.

STEP 5: DIFFERENT STROKES FOR DIFFERENT FOLKS

The CAP and PLS provided more structure than the tactual and kinesthetic (movement oriented) resources, but it was amazing how some students were drawn to one and not the other. When students who require structure are asked to break their routine, they often feel uneasy. Some enjoyed every resource; some preferred one very much more than others; some asked to experience each before deciding; two or three asked if I intended to ever lecture again! (How good to be needed!)

Some students worked at their desks; others chose to sit on the floor. Some worked in brightly lit window areas; others migrated toward softly lit sections of the room. A few moved into the adjacent hall but worked there diligently. Some worked alone, others in pairs, others in a small cooperative group; still others became competitive in teams, and a few remained close to my side.

We have all seen these different types of students, but in the past, we have ignored their differences. My professor's learning-style resources acknowledged and responded to their differences. And this teacher—with five years' worth of experience—learned an awful lot that first day, just by watching my students' reactions and listening to their comments.

STEP 6: RECOGNIZING GLOBAL VERSUS ANALYTIC LEARNERS

The Dunns (1993) describe global learners as people who first need to understand how a concept relates to them and their lives before they can concentrate on details and facts. Being the opposite, an analytic, I have always taught details and facts first, gradually building up to an understanding of a topic. It was most astonishing to see these two types of learners emerge as my students used the various global and analytic resources. Somehow, they knew immediately if what they were using worked for them. They began asking why some of them learned quickly with one resource and others learned better with a different resource. We lapsed into conversations about the differences among how perfectly able people learn new and difficult information.

Those of us in nursing know that much of what we have been taught has been introduced in small steps sequentially (analytically). However, remember the nursing students who flourished in the clinical work but struggled with the facts? Remember the ones who were great when memorizing facts and then were clueless in the labs? What more evidence do we need to soberly introduce learning-style-based instruction than that we have at least these two types of learners in every class and, whatever our style, we are responding to only one group!

STEP 7: ASSUMING RESPONSIBILITY FOR THEIR OWN LEARNING

Students asked if they could take my materials home to study, but I needed to show and report on their use to my professor! Instead, I offered to teach them how to make the materials of their choice for their own home use, and they immediately responded enthusiastically. Some said that they would study other subjects this way. Two students graciously asked when I planned to resume lecturing. I, equally graciously, ignored the groan emitted by many of the others present.

STEP 8: LEARNING BEYOND ACADEMICS

Here's what happened in that class: Most of my students seemed to intuit their own learning-style preferences. They just had never understood that the way they learned was acceptable. They certainly had never known how to help themselves master new and difficult material other than through reading the text, rereading their notes, and trying to guess what was going to be on the exams.

They weren't familiar with any of the labels—global, analytic, impulsive, reflective, structure, and so forth—but each had struggled with certain content repeatedly. They certainly had preconceived erroneous ideas about "right" and "wrong" ways to study, and they hadn't known that, whatever their style, it was acceptable if they knew how to make it work for them.

Some had felt "stupid" because they couldn't remember a lot of what their teachers had lectured about. Others couldn't take notes in class; they couldn't quite figure out what was so important that it ought to be written. Several had been chastised because they fiddled and doodled while listening, never realizing that they were tactual and/or global. Others had been admonished to "sit up and pay attention" and had not known that they needed an informal design and either tactual or kinesthetic, rather than auditory resources. Slowly their confidence began to surface, and several actually verbalized that they now felt that they *could* succeed.

Toward the end of the semester, I tested students with the Productivity Environmental Preference Survey (PEPS) (Dunn & Dunn, 1972). Next semester I'll give each student a printed prescription for studying and doing their homework through their learning-style strengths (Dunn

& Klavas, 1987). I showed them how to create many of their own study materials, and they did that on their own time. And, from that very first unit on the heart, my students began achieving better than they did before and were thoroughly enjoying learning.

Eventually they shared their wonder at how much they were actually learning from the floor game and the tactual manipulatives. Many showed classmates in other classes and at their jobs how to teach themselves with their preferred resources. Since this particular population was fairly independent to begin with, they enjoyed choosing how they would learn in class—alone, in pairs, in small groups, or sometimes by questioning me. They liked the feeling of being able to control their own learning and, better still, they accepted total responsibility for teaching themselves.

Most students reported that learning about the cardiovascular system actually became easier as they increasingly involved themselves in mastering the objectives, each in his or her own way. Not one ever complained that I hadn't "covered" anything. No one whined about forthcoming tests! Confidence increased as they compared their knowledge and tried to anticipate what would be on each test! Test scores were the highest I had ever seen on that unit in any class! And the halls were buzzing with the excitement of what was happening in my class.

STEP 9: NATURAL OUTCOMES

Other professors asked me to explain what I was doing. I left all the materials in either the resource center or in my office for interested students and colleagues. Students who moved into other units returned to the heart materials for review and to duplicate the resources for the following unit that we were then studying.

The CAP and the PLS were seen as a "gift from God" by my analytics; the floor game and tactual resources were repeatedly blessed by my globals—many of whom also enjoyed the PLS. Before long, I was serving as a guide to their instruction; the resources themselves were doing the teaching, and the students were actively involved in teaching themselves or each other.

After a short time, a kind of competition began. Students began to time the completion of CAPs and PLSs. They were moving through units at a faster rate than I believed possible, and I feared that their learning was only superficial. Not true. Test scores continued to soar, and by the end of the semester, each unit they studied revealed better scores than I had seen during my five years of teaching. Not only that, the fear of tests seemed to dissipate. They were eager to demonstrate how much they had learned and some said that they no longer had to "really study" for the test. Everything they had learned was retained.

STEP 10: PLANNING FOR NEXT SEMESTER

In addition to the improved grades, it was refreshing to see students proud and happy about their accomplishments. I have promised myself to make administration of the PEPS part of every syllabus I use from now on. It didn't really take a lot of effort—just courage. I've already shared my decision with colleagues. Several professors were really positive about the test results I saw and want to try learning styles. Others are as fearful as I was. I've encouraged them because I now have visions of the students demonstrating incredible results on the state licensing examinations. I'm confident about *my* students' scores.

STEP 11: ENCOURAGING COLLEAGUES

We, in nursing, need to do more than merely pay lip service to individual differences. Nothing works for students like this model of learning styles, and it's relatively easy to implement. After my initial personal trauma, my students did most of the work, and they thanked me for teaching them how to succeed.

Once the connection between learning styles and examination scores becomes evident, you will not want to stop. Our nursing students take so many multiple-choice examinations that it should be relatively easy to determine how much learning style contributes to their increased achievement. Consider how learning styles could improve clinical performance. Analytics, who are best at memorizing, could focus on the procedures first, then practice, and then take the test, whereas globals could observe and assist in the lab by practicing the skills and then focus on each of the steps prior to the test. Just using the right sequence for different learners might be an answer to improved performance.

If you remain hesitant, read a couple of articles that really impressed me (Griggs, Griggs, Dunn, & Ingham, 1994; Lenehan et al., 1994). If that research doesn't convince you, I recommend that you apply for admission into the doctoral program in which I currently am a student. Once involved, Old Brick-Wall will see that you get started—and you'll succeed as well, or better, than I.

Epilogue

Suggested Future Directions

Rita Dunn

Shirley A. Griggs

If you found this book on learning styles interesting, you may want additional information. Since 1979, St. John's University's Center for the Study of Learning and Teaching Styles (CSLTS) has been actively engaged in conducting research, distributing information, developing and publishing resources, and providing staff development for people and organizations concerned with the practical applications of learning-style approaches.

Each July, CSLTS conducts a one-week Leadership Certification Institute on learning styles in New York City. Persons who attend and complete all requirements can be certified as a Learning-Styles Trainer. If you are interested, contact Professor Rita Dunn, Director, CLSTS, St. John's University, New York 11439, and request a free brochure.

During the past two decades, an international learning-styles network of researchers and practitioners has emerged to assist others in becoming knowledgeable about their learning styles (see table on page 99). Network members believe the following:

1. Each person is unique, can learn, and has an individual learning style.

2. Individual learning styles should be acknowledged and respected.

3. Learning style is a function of heredity and experience, including strengths and limitations, and develops individually over each person's life span.

4. Learning style is a combination of affective, cognitive, environmental, and physiological responses that characterize how a person learns.

97

5. Individual information processing is fundamental to a learning style and can be strengthened over time with intervention.

6. Learning style is a complex construct for which a comprehensive understanding is evolving.

7. Learners are empowered by a knowledge of their own and others' learning styles.

8. Effective curriculum and instruction are learning style-based and personalized to address and honor diversity.

9. Effective teachers continually monitor activities to ensure compatibility of instruction and evaluation with each individual's learning-style strengths.

10. Teaching individuals through their learning-style strengths improves their achievement, self-esteem, and attitude toward learning.

11. Each individual is entitled to counseling and instruction that respond to his or her style of learning.

12. A viable learning-style model must be grounded in theoretical and applied research, periodically evaluated, and adapted to reflect the developing knowledge base.

13. Implementation of learning-style practices must adhere to accepted standards of professional ethics.

International Learning Style Network Centers

Institutions	Locations	Directors
Alabama A & M	Huntsville, AL	Dr. Annie Wells
Aquinas College	Grand Rapids, MI	Dr. Katy Lux and Mrs. Connie Bouwman
Center for Creative Learning	Sarasota, FL	Dr. Donald Treffinger
Dowling College	Oakdale, NY	Dr. Bernadyn Suh and Dr. Thomas C. DeBello
ERIE 1 Board of Cooperative Educational Services	Buffalo, NY	Pam Giambalucca
George Mason University and Fairfax County School District	Fairfax, VA	Dr. Barbara Given and Mrs. Linda Clark
Lon Morris College	Jacksonville, TX	Mrs. Sherrye Dotson
Marckwort Business Association	Helsinki, Finland	Mr. and Mrs. Auvo and Raya Marckwort
College of Christchurch	New Zealand	Dr. Alan C. Webster
North Carolina Teacher Academy	Durham, NC	Mrs. Julia Kron
Ohio State University	Columbus, OH	Dr. Barbara Thomson
The Philippines' Learning Styles Center	Manila, The Philippines	Mr. Henry Tendero
St. John's University	Jamaica, NY	Dr. Rita Dunn
Tarleton State University	Texas	Dr. Pam Littleton and Dr. Janet Valdez
University of South Carolina–Aiken	Aiken, SC	Dr. Margaret Riedell and Dr. Alice Sheehan
Performance Concepts International, Ltd.	Pittsford, NY	Susan Rundle and Tina Simpson

References

Anderson, J. (1988). Cognitive styles and multicultural populations. *Journal of Teacher Education, 39*(1), 2–9.

Beaty, S. A. (1986). The effect of inservice training on the ability of teachers to observe learning styles of students (Doctoral Dissertation, Oregon State University). *Dissertation Abstracts International, 47,* 1988A.

Billings, D., & Cobb, K. (1992). Effects of learning style preference, attitude, and GPA on learner achievement using computer-assisted-interactive videodisc instruction. *Journal of Computer-Based Instruction, 19*(1), 12–16.

Bratt, E., & Vockell, E. (1986, June). Using computers to teach basic facts in the nursing curriculum. *Journal of Nursing Education, 25*(6), 247–250.

Brennan, P. K. (1984). An analysis of the relationships among hemispheric preference and analytic/global cognitive style, two elements of learning style, method of instruction, gender, and mathematics achievement of tenth-grade geometry students (Doctoral dissertation, St. John's University, 1984). *Dissertation Abstracts International, 45,* 3271A.

Buell, B. G., & Buell, N. A. (1987). Perceptual modality preference as a variable in the effectiveness of continuing education for professionals (Doctoral Dissertation, University of Southern California, 1987). *Dissertation Abstracts International, 48,* 23A.

Caine, R. N., & Caine, G. (1991). *Making connections: Teaching and the human brain.* Alexandria, VA: Association for Supervision and Curriculum Development.

101

Canfield, A. A., & Lafferty, J. C. (1976). *Learning Style Inventory*. Detroit: Humanics Media.

Clark-Thayer, S. (1987). The relationship of the knowledge of student-perceived learning style preferences, and study habits and attitudes to achievement of college freshmen in a small urban university (Doctoral dissertation, Boston University, 1987). *Dissertation Abstracts International, 48,* 872A.

Clark-Thayer, S. (1988). Designing study-skills programs based on individual learning-styles. *Learning-Style Network Newsletter, 9*(3), 4.

Claxton, C. S., & Murrell, P. H. (1987). *Learning styles: Implications for improving education practices* (ASHE-ERIC Higher Education Report No. 4). Washington, DC: Association for the Study of Higher Education.

Cody, C. (1983). Learning styles, including hemispheric dominance: A comparative study of average, gifted, and highly gifted students in grades five through twelve (Doctoral dissertation, Temple University, 1983). *Dissertation Abstracts International, 44,* 1631A.

Coleman, S. J. (1988). An investigation of the relationships among physical and emotional learning style preferences and perceptual modality strengths of gifted first-grade students (Doctoral dissertation, Virginia Polytechnic Institute and State University, 1988). *Dissertation Abstracts International, 50*(04), 873A.

Cook, L. (1989). Relationships among learning style awareness, academic achievement, and locus of control among community college students (Doctoral dissertation, University of Florida, 1989). *Dissertation Abstracts International, 49*(03), 217A.

Cross, J. A. (1982). Internal locus of control governs talented students (−12). *Learning Styles Network Newsletter, 3*(3), 3.

Curry, L. (1987). *Integrating concepts of cognitive or learning styles: A review with attention to psychometric standards.* Ottawa, Ontario: Canadian College of Health Services Executives.

DeBello, T. (1990, July–September). Comparison of eleven major learning styles models: Variables, appropriate populations, validity of instrumentation, and the research behind them. *Journal of Reading, Writing, and Learning Disabilities International, 6*(3), 203–222.

DeCoux, V. H. (1990). Kolb's Learning Style Inventory: A review of its application in nursing research. *Journal of Nursing Education, 29*(5), 202–207.

Douglas, C. B. (1979). Making biology easier to understand. *The Biology Teacher, 4*(50), 277–299.

Dunn, R. (1987). Research on instructional environments: Implications for student achievement and results. *Professional School Psychology, 2*(1), 43–52.

Dunn, R. (1989, Fall). Teaching gifted students through their learning style strengths. *International Education, 16*(51), 6–8.

Dunn, R. (1990). Understanding the Dunn and Dunn Learning Styles Model and the need for individual diagnosis and prescription. *Reading, Writing, and Learning Disabilities International, 6,* 223–247.

Dunn, R. (1992). Strategies for teaching word recognition to disabled readers. *Reading and Writing Quarterly: Overcoming Learning Difficulties, 8,* 157–177.

Dunn, R. (1996). *How to implement and supervise a learning style program.* Alexandria, VA: Association for Supervision and Curriculum Development.

Dunn, R., Bruno, J., Sklar, R. I., Zenhausern, R., & Beaudry, J. (1990, May/June). Effects of matching and mismatching minority developmental college students' hemispheric preferences on mathematics scores. *Journal of Educational Research, 83*(5), 283–288.

Dunn, R., Cavanaugh, D., Eberle, B., & Zenhausern, R. (1982). Hemispheric preference: The newest element of learning style. *The American Biology Teacher, 44*(5), 291–294.

Dunn, R., DeBello, T., Brennan, P., Krimsky, J., & Murrain, P. (1981). Learning style researchers define differences differently. *Educational Leadership, 38*(5), 382–392.

Dunn, R., Deckinger, E. L., Withers, P., & Katzenstein, H. (1990, Winter). Should college students be taught how to do homework? The effects of studying marketing through individual perceptual strengths. *Illinois School Research and Development Journal, 26*(3), 96–113.

Dunn, R., & Dunn, K. (1972). *Practical approaches to individualizing instruction: Contracts and other effective teaching strategies.* Nyack, New York: Parker/Prentice-Hall.

Dunn, R., & Dunn, K. (1975). *Educator's self-teaching guide to individualizing instructional programs.* Nyack, NY: Parker/Prentice-Hall.

Dunn, R., & Dunn, K. (1978). *Teaching students through their individual learning styles: A practical approach.* Reston, Virginia: Reston/Prentice-Hall.

Dunn, R., & Dunn, K. (1992). *Teaching elementary students through their individual learning styles: Practical approaches for grades 3–6.* Boston: Allyn & Bacon.

Dunn, R., & Dunn, K. (1993). *Teaching secondary students through their individual learning styles: Practical approaches for grades 7–12.* Boston: Allyn & Bacon.

Dunn, R., Dunn, K., & Price, G. E. (1982/1989). *Productivity Environmental Preference Survey.* Lawrence, KS: Price Systems.

Dunn, R., Dunn, K., & Price, G. E. (1989). *Learning Style Inventory.* Lawrence, KS: Price Systems.

Dunn, R., Dunn, K., & Treffinger, D. (1992). *Bringing out the giftedness in every child: A guide for parents.* New York: Wiley.

Dunn, R., & Griggs, S. A. (1995). *Multiculturalism and learning styles: Teaching and counseling adolescents.* Westport, CT: Greenwood Press.

Dunn, R., Griggs, S. A., Olson, J., Gorman, B., & Beasley, M. (1995). A meta analytic validation of the Dunn and Dunn learning styles model. *Journal of Educational Research, 88*(6), 353–361.

Dunn, R., & Klavas, A. (1990). *Homework disc: How to study and do homework based on individual learning style strengths.* Jamaica, NY: St. John's University's Center for the Study of Learning and Teaching Styles.

Dunn, R., & Milgram, R. (1993). Learning styles and gifted students in diverse cultures. In R. M. Milgram, R. Dunn, & G. E. Price (Eds.), *Teaching and counseling gifted and talented adolescents: An international learning style perspective* (pp. 3–23). Westport, CT: Praeger.

Dunn, R., & Price, G. E. (1980). The learning style characteristics of gifted children. *Gifted Child Quarterly, 24*(1), 33–36.

Dunn, R., Sklar, R. I., Beaudry, J. S., & Bruno, J. (1990). Effects of matching and mismatching minority developmental college students' hemispheric preferences on mathematics scores. *Journal of Educational Research, 83*(5), 283–288.

Freeley, M. E., & Perrin, J. (1987, August/September). Teaching to both hemispheres. *Teaching K–8,* 67–69.

Gregorc, A. R. (1982). *Style delineator.* Maynard, MA: Gabriel Systems.

Griggs, D., Griggs, S. A., Dunn, R., & Ingham, J. (1994). A challenge for nurse educators: Accommodating nursing students' diverse learning styles. *Nurse Educator, 19*(6), 41–45.

Griggs, S. A. (1993, Autumn). Suggestions for future research in the health professions. *Learning Styles Network Newsletter, 14*(2), 4.

Griggs, S. A., & Price, G. E. (1980). A comparison between the learning styles of gifted versus average junior high school students. *Phi Delta Kappan, 61,* 361.

Hancock, V. (1995). Information literacy, brain-based learning, and the technological revolution. *School Library Media Activities Monthly, 12*(1), 31–34.

Hill, J. (1971). *Personalized education programs: Utilizing cognitive style mapping.* Bloomfield Hills, MI: Oakland Community College.

Huffman, E. (1994). *Health information management.* Berwyn, IL: Physicians' Record.

Ingham, J. (1991). Matching instruction with employee perceptual preferences significantly increases training effectiveness. *Human Resource Development Quarterly, 2*(1), 53–64.

Jarsonbeck, S. (1984). The effects of a right-brain and mathematics curriculum on low achieving, fourth grade students (Doctoral dissertation, University of South Florida, 1984). *Dissertation Abstracts International, 45,* 2791A.

Keefe, J. W. (1982). Foreword. In *Student learning styles and brain behavior.* Reston, VA: National Association of Secondary School Principals.

Keefe, J. W., Languis, M., Letteri, C., & Dunn, R. (1986). *Learning style profile.* Reston, VA: National Association of Secondary School Principals.

Khoiny, F. E. (1995, July/August). Factors that contribute to computer-assisted instruction effectiveness. *Computers in Nursing, 13*(4), 165–168.

Kirby, P. (1979). *Cognitive style, learning style, and transfer skill acquisition.* Columbus, OH: Ohio State University, National Center for Research in Vocational Education.

Koch, E. W., Rankin, J. A., & Stewart, R. (1990, March). Nursing students' preferences in the use of computer-assisted learning. *Journal of Nursing Education, 29*(3), 122–126.

Kolb, D. A. (1976). *Learning Style Inventory.* Boston: McBer.

Kreitner, K. R. (1981). *Modality strengths and learning styles of musically talented high school students.* Unpublished master's dissertation, Ohio State University, Columbus.

LaMothe, J., Billings, D. M., Belcher, A., Cobb, K., Nice, A., & Richardson, V. (1991). Reliability and validity of the Productivity Environmental Preference Survey (PEPS). *Nurse Educator, 16*(4), 30–35.

Lan Yong, F. (1989). *Ethnic, gender, and grade differences in the learning style preferences of gifted minority students.* Unpublished doctoral dissertation, Southern Illinois University, Carbondale.

Laschinger, H. K., & Bass, M. W. (1984). Learning styles of nursing students and career choice. *Journal of Advanced Nursing, 9,* 375–380.

Lenehan, M. C., Dunn, R., Ingham, J., Murray, W., & Signer, B. (1994, November). Learning style: Necessary know-how for academic success in college. *Journal of College Student Development, 35,* 461–466.

Letteri, C. (1985). Teaching students how to learn. *Theory into Practice, 24,* 112–122.

Marcus, L. (1977). A comparison of selected ninth-grade male and female students' learning styles. *The Journal, 6*(3), 27–28.

Matson, G. D. (1980). Modifying the impulsive cognitive learning style by instructional materials and teacher modeling (Doctoral dissertation, Florida State University, 1980). *Dissertation Abstracts International, 41*(052), 1872A.

Mein, J. R. (1986). Cognitive and learning style characteristics of high school gifted students (Doctoral dissertation, University of Florida, 1986). *Dissertation Abstracts International, 48*(04), 880A.

Mickler, M. L., & Zippert, C. P. (1987). Teaching strategies based on learning styles of adult students. *Community/Junior College Quarterly, 11,* 33–37.

Milgram, R. M., Dunn, R., & Price, G. E. (Eds.). (1993). *Teaching and counseling gifted and talented adolescents for learning style: An international perspective.* Westport: CT: Greenwood Press.

Miller, J. (1997). *Effects of traditional versus learning-style presentations of course content in ultrasound and anatomy on the achievement and attitudes of college students.* Doctoral dissertation, St. John's University, Jamaica, NY.

Myers, I. (1962). *Myers-Briggs Type Indicator.* Palo-Alto, CA: Consulting Psychologists Press.

Nelson, B., Dunn, R., Griggs, S. A., Primavera, L., Fitzpatrick, M., & Miller, R. (1993, September). Effects of learning style intervention on college students' retention and achievement. *Journal of College Student Development, 34*(5), 364–369.

O'Keefe, J., & Nadel, L. (1978). *The Hippocampus as a cognitive map.* Oxford, MA: Clarendon Press.

Orenstein, R., & Sobel, D. (1987). *The healing brain.* New York: Simon & Schuster.

Paskewitz, B. U. (1985). A study of the relationship between learning styles and attitudes toward computer programming of middle school gifted students (Doctoral dissertation, University of Pittsburgh, 1985). *Dissertation Abstracts International, 47*(03), 697A.

Pederson, J. K. (1984). The classification and comparison of learning disabled students and gifted students (Doctoral dissertation, Texas Tech University, 1984). *Dissertation Abstracts International, 45*(09A), 2810.

Perrin, J. (1984). An experimental investigation of the relationships among the learning style sociological preferences of gifted and nongifted primary children, selected instructional strategies, attitudes, and achievement in problem solving and rote memorization (Doctoral dissertation, St. John's University, 1984). *Dissertation Abstracts International, 46*, 342A.

Perrin, J. (1990, October). The learning styles project for potential dropouts. *Educational Leadership, 48*(2), 23–24.

Pizzo, J., Dunn, R., & Dunn, K. (1990, July/September). A sound approach to reading: Responding to students' learning styles. *Journal of Reading, Writing, and Learning Disabilities International, 6*(3), 249–260.

Price, G. E. (1980). Which learning style elements are stable and which tend to change over time? *Learning Styles Network Newsletter, 1*(3), 1.

Price, G. E., Dunn, K., Dunn, R., & Griggs, S. A. (1981). Studies in students' learning styles. *Roeper Review, 4*, 223–226.

Ramirez, M., & Castenada, A. (1974). *Cultural democracy, bicognitive development, and education.* New York: Academic Press.

Research on the Dunn and Dunn Model. (1997). Jamaica, NY: St. John's University's Center for the Study of Learning and Teaching Styles.

Restak, R. (1979). *The brain: The last frontier.* Garden City, NY: Doubleday.

Ricca, J. (1983). Curricular implications of learning style differences between gifted and non-gifted students (Doctoral dissertation, State University of New York at Buffalo, 1983). *Dissertation Abstracts International, 44,* 1324-A.

St. John's University, Center for the Study of Learning and Teaching Styles. (1997). *Articles & Books.* Jamaica, NY: Author.

Schmeck, R. R. (1977). *Inventory of learning processes.* Carbondale: Department of Psychology, Southern Illinois University.

Spielberger, C. D., Barker, L., Russell, S., DeCrane, S., Westberry, L., Knight, J., & Marks, E. (1979). *Preliminary manual for the State-Trait Personality Inventory.* Tampa: University of South Florida.

Springer, S., & Deutsch, G. (1985). *Left brain, right brain.* New York: Freeman.

Stewart, E. D. (1981). Learning styles among gifted/talented students: Instructional technique preferences. *Exceptional Children, 48,* 113–138.

Stone, Pete. (1992, November). How we turned around a problem school. *The Principal, 71*(2), 34–36.

Sullivan, M. (1993). A meta-analysis of experimental research studies based on the Dunn and Dunn learning styles model and its relationship to academic achievement and performance (Doctoral dissertation, St. John's University, 1993). *Dissertation Abstracts International, 51*(98), 2976.

Sylwester, R. (1995). *A celebration of neurons: An educator's guide to the human brain.* Alexandria, VA: Association for Supervision and Curriculum Development.

Tannenbaum, R. (1982). An investigation of the relationships between selected instructional techniques and identified field dependent and field independent cognitive styles as evidenced among high school students enrolled in studies of nutrition (Doctoral dissertation, St. John's University, 1982). *Dissertation Abstracts International, 43,* 63A.

Thies, A. (1995/July). *The decade of the brain.* Presentation at the 19th annual Learning Styles Institute sponsored by St. John's University, New York.

Thies, A. P. (1979). A brain behavior analysis of learning style. In *Student learning styles: Diagnosing and prescribing programs.* Reston, VA: National Association of Secondary School Principals.

Vignia, R. A. (1983). An investigation of learning styles of gifted and non-gifted high school students (Doctoral dissertation, University of Houston, 1983). *Dissertation Abstracts International, 44,* 3653A.

Wasson, F. (1980). *A comparative analysis of learning style and personality characteristics of achieving and underachieving gifted elementary students.* Unpublished doctoral dissertation, Florida State University.

Witkin, H. A., Oltman, P., Raskin, E., & Karp, S. A. (1971). *Embedded Figures Test.* Palo Alto, CA: Consulting Psychologists Press.

Zenhausern, R. (1980). Hemispheric dominance. *Learning Styles Network Newsletter, 2*(3).

Index